# Detox Memoir

Dr. Christopher J. Dorais

Copyright © 2014 Dr. Christopher J. Dorais
All rights reserved.

ISBN: 1500854549
ISBN 13: 9781500854546
Library of Congress Control Number: 2014914792
CreateSpace Independent Publishing Platform
North Charleston, South Carolina

"My people perish for a lack of knowledge."

~Hosea 4:6

# Introduction

This book will *not* change your life. Yes, you read that correctly. In a world where "change your life" claims are made concerning a great many things, I would like this book to stand in stark contrast to all of that. God can change your life. You can change your life. This book cannot. This is not a science book, nor is it a medical textbook on detoxification. I am not a medical doctor, nor do I give medical advice in this book. I do have a doctoral degree, but it's not in medicine—it's in education. And that is what this memoir will give you—an education.

*Detox Memoir* chronicles my twelve-year journey from sickness to health. Like any memoir, it contains some very personal information. These personal details were necessary because I wanted to tell you the truth—all of it. Even if this truth is at times embarrassing or unpleasant, you are going to hear it all.

Because this book is a memoir, you will find that much of the writing is very conversational. Please don't equate my conversational style as an indicator of the accuracy, or lack thereof, of the scientific concepts presented here. I have attempted to back up most of my claims and theories with solid peer-reviewed scientific research, cited in the reference section. But I don't always cite my sources. Some of my ideas came from a website or blog that made just a passing reference to a certain idea I was considering, so these would be fairly pointless to reference. Sometimes I just went forward with a detox theory or protocol based upon faith, intuition, and good, old-fashioned, science speculation. This is just one of the many reasons why this book cannot be considered a research book. It is only what it claims to be: a memoir of one person's health changes over a twelve-year period.

Maybe you are reading this book because you are sick. Perhaps you are seriously ill. More likely however, you are just feeling a bit out of sorts. Something is not quite right. You don't feel the way you used to. Old age seems to have snuck up on you suddenly, and you are looking for answers as to why this happened. "All of a sudden, my body just seems to be falling apart!" I know this feeling very well. That person was me over twelve years ago.

If you live on this planet, you will have health problems sooner or later. Every person eventually becomes a patient. It is my personal opinion that most people develop health problems due to toxicity in their environment. All people are exposed to toxins, whether from the food we eat, the water we drink, or the air we breathe. We even produce our own toxins internally. All of these toxins cause a great deal of sickness because they increase our vulnerability to the harmful fungi, bacteria, and viruses around us, and in us.

Sometimes we take medicines to alleviate some of the conditions caused by toxicity. The irony of this is that many medicines are also toxic. Do you doubt this? Let me ask you this question: have you ever read a list of side effects on a prescription bottle? What about the long list of potential side effects rapidly spoken by the narrator of that TV commercial for a prescription drug? Side effects occur because of toxicity! In short, we are all toxic. The only difference between us is our degree of toxicity.

Some of what you will read in this memoir may sound incredible, perhaps even unbelievable. Memoirs tend to be that way. It's one reason why I am not making any claims for wellness or promises of healing. If, by reading this memoir, you get some ideas or inspiration that you feel may help you in your own situation, then *Detox Memoir* has served a good purpose. I believe every step taken that contributed to my improving health was completely science-based, but I cannot offer any proof of this apart from my own results. My goal from the onset was to test theories and protocols on myself to see if I could get better. I conducted many experiments, but not in a manner that would qualify them as truly scientific. There was no large pool of subjects being used in a double-blind experiment. There was usually just me, and the results are the story you are about to read.

My challenge to you as the reader is to seek out the evidence for yourself. I have found that only when people research questionable claims on their

## INTRODUCTION

own, particularly when the subject is health and wellness, do they truly believe what they are reading. It's only when you truly believe something that you will take ownership of that knowledge and act on it. And only when you act on something will real and lasting change come into your life. So as you read through this memoir and you start to question some of my tactics, strategy, or logic, I urge you to do the research on your own. If you approach the research with an open mind, you might be very surprised with what you find.

I do not know your particular situation, but I do know mine. I was sick—now I am well. Over a decade ago, my body and my life were falling apart. Now, both my body and my life have been built up again. I have recovered all of those years lost to sickness. This is my story as to what I believe caused my sickness, and what paths I took to regain my health. This is my personal detox story, and perhaps someday, it may be yours as well.

# Dedication

I dedicate this book to anyone who is sick without a *known* cause. That person was me. One day, I was perfectly healthy—or so I thought—and the very next day, I found myself in the miserable world of "sickness unknown." I tried modern allopathic medicine for about five years and basically found nothing but disappointment and debt. For the next seven years, with the help of homeopathic doctors and detoxification experts, I put together my own wellness plan. Although I experienced far more failures than successes along the way, I finally found a way through the smoke and fog of sickness unknown. If this is your current situation, where you are sick and feel totally lost, I know personally the wretched frustration you undoubtedly feel. At times, the pain and distress seem almost unbearable. You have tried doctors with reputations high and low, paid out-of-pocket expenses for treatments that seemed questionable, and have taken nutritional supplements by the handfuls, only to see little if any improvement in your condition. It is my desire that this book will provide you with hope and help, which will gradually evolve into a workable plan that will lead you back to health and wellness.

This memoir is based largely on a journal that I kept as I was searching for answers to my health problems. If, in the reading of this memoir, you find it tedious in terms of seemingly irrelevant details, there is a reason for this. I wanted you as the reader to walk the path that I did. I wanted you to understand what I felt, especially in the early years of my story, when I really had no idea what was going on. All of these details were necessary in order to paint a complete picture of my condition and experiences. As you work your way through this memoir, I have little doubt you will ask yourself if what worked for me will work for you. I cannot answer this question. My detox protocols worked wonderfully well *for me*. But I can offer you no guarantee concerning your own condition. Each person has a unique genetic signature, and therefore, each person may have a slightly different response to toxicity and to detox protocols. But toxicities do have very strong commonalities, both in symptoms and in treatment. My prayer is that if you have a toxicity problem—and most people do—my story may be of great help to you as you make your own way from sickness, to renewed vitality and robust health.

Disclaimer

THE CONTENTS OF THIS BOOK ARE FOR EDUCATIONAL AND INFORMATIONAL PURPOSES ONLY. NEITHER THE AUTHOR NOR THE PUBLISHER IS ENGAGED IN RENDERING PROFESSIONAL MEDICAL ADVICE OR MEDICAL SERVICES TO THE READER. THIS BOOK IS NOT MEANT TO BE **MEDICAL ADVICE**, NOR IS IT A **PRESCRIPTION** FOR ANY ILLNESS OR CONDITION. THE AUTHOR AND THE PUBLISHER ARE NOT LIABLE OR RESPONSIBLE FOR ANY LOSS, INJURY, OR DAMAGE ALLEGEDLY ARISING FROM ANY INFORMATION OR SUGGESTION IN THIS BOOK. THE AUTHOR AND THE PUBLISHER ARE ABSOLVED OF ANY RESPONSIBILITY ARISING FROM ANY USE OF THIS INFORMATION.

THESE STATEMENTS ARE TO BE CONSIDERED DISCLAIMERS OF RESPONSIBILITY FOR ANYTHING PUBLISHED HERE. THE AUTHOR AND PUBLISHER PROVIDE THE INFORMATION IN THIS BOOK WITH THE UNDERSTANDING THAT YOU MAY ACT ON IT AT YOUR OWN RISK AND ALSO WITH THE FULL KNOWLEDGE THAT HEALTH PROFESSIONALS SHOULD ALWAYS BE CONSULTED FIRST BEFORE ANY ACTION IS TAKEN. YOU SHOULD FIRST CONSULT WITH A PHYSICIAN WHO IS KNOWLEDGEABLE AND TRAINED IN ALTERNATIVE AND NATURAL HEALING MODALITIES TO DETERMINE WHETHER ANY OF THE PROTOCOLS AND PROCEDURES DISCUSSED IN THIS BOOK WORK, OR WHETHER THEY ARE OF ANY VALUE.

# Table of Contents

| | | |
|---|---|---|
| Chapter 1: | Sickness Unknown | 1 |
| Chapter 2: | Looking for Causes in All the Wrong Places | 5 |
| Chapter 3: | A New Level of Weird | 10 |
| Chapter 4: | Please Pass the Snake Oil | 16 |
| Chapter 5: | A Slight Paradigm Shift | 20 |
| Chapter 6: | Asking the Right Questions | 29 |
| Chapter 7: | Not Eating "Just Anything" Anymore | 40 |
| Chapter 8: | By Any Other Name | 43 |
| Chapter 9: | Taking Stock and Getting Stretched | 47 |
| Chapter 10: | Clues from a Close Shave | 52 |
| Chapter 11: | Too Much Trust | 55 |
| Chapter 12: | Frailty, Thy Name Is Mercury | 61 |
| Chapter 13: | Skeptical Yet? | 67 |
| Chapter 14: | Plotting a Course | 71 |
| Chapter 15: | Taking that First Step | 79 |
| Chapter 16: | Skin for Skin | 86 |
| Chapter 17: | Under Mike's Drill | 89 |
| Chapter 18: | The Look | 91 |
| Chapter 19: | The Terrifying Theoretical Leap | 95 |
| Chapter 20: | Light the Fuse | 103 |
| Chapter 21: | Breaking Through | 108 |
| Chapter 22: | The New Plan | 116 |
| Chapter 23: | One Very Interesting Year | 123 |
| Chapter 24: | The Undiplomatic Breakthrough | 128 |
| Chapter 25: | Fog | 135 |
| Chapter 26: | What Comes Out Goes Around | 143 |
| Chapter 27: | Crisis of Healing | 146 |
| Chapter 28: | A New Sensitivity | 152 |

| | | |
|---|---|---|
| Chapter 29: | Human Canary | 156 |
| Chapter 30: | An Ancient Remedy | 161 |
| Chapter 31: | The Unexpected Hormonal Connection | 167 |
| Chapter 32: | Convergence | 172 |
| Chapter 33: | Thyroid Reboot | 180 |
| Chapter 34: | The Supplanting Agents | 187 |
| Chapter 35: | Predictability | 196 |
| Chapter 36: | Not a Chance | 201 |
| Chapter 37: | Different Problem, Same Solution | 206 |
| Chapter 38: | Dipping Seven Times in the Jordan | 210 |
| Chapter 39: | From Symbiotic to Parasitic | 223 |
| Chapter 40: | Welcome to Your Life | 238 |
| Epilogue | | 251 |

# Chapter 1

# Sickness Unknown

My sickness came to my attention over twelve years ago, but I have no doubt that these problems actually began before I was born. In fact, I believe my toxicity problems began before my mother was born as well. I believe that most of my health problems were passed down through the generations, starting perhaps with my maternal great-grandmother. How can such a thing even be possible? To answer this question, it is better that I tell you my story, and then perhaps this statement will make sense.

I grew up in Michigan, in a climate with four full seasons, and my overall health was, for as long as I can remember, just a little above average. I seemed to always fall victim to Michigan's seasonal colds and flus. Typically, my bouts with sickness would last for about two weeks, and though they varied in severity from year to year, I could expect to fall victim to some sort of illness every year. Unfortunately, I did not grow out of my proclivity to seasonal sicknesses—I carried it with me into my adult life. I am a teacher by trade, and as the students began coughing and sneezing in the fall, it was just a matter of time before I would do the same.

Aside from this seasonal sickness problem, thankfully, I have never been seriously ill. I considered myself health conscious, but really this was only in reference to exercise. When it came to my diet, I freely admit that I often made very poor choices with what I ate. I didn't really consider junk food, junk food until it upset my stomach. Like most people, I loved to eat sweets, and I drank more than just my fair share of soft drinks. The funny thing is, if you would have asked me back in those days if I thought that I was taking good care of my body, I would have said yes. After all, I didn't smoke tobacco or drink alcohol, and I exercised regularly. True, I had a penchant for fast food, but it wasn't like I ate out every day. I was also very active in sports, and that kept me in fairly good physical condition. Looking back, it is somewhat ironic that it was my performance in sports that began to reveal early signs of toxicity damage, though of course, I didn't know it at the time.

I have played sports my whole life. As such, I have experienced the same sports-related aches and pains that any athlete does. Without a doubt, my favorite sport was basketball. I have played competitive basketball since the third grade, but by my mid-twenties, my ability to play the game started to diminish because of weakness in my lower back. It was frequently sore and often required ice after most rigorous activities, with the exception of swimming. But like most people who are young and active, I ignored the pain, used ice when I needed it, and moved on with my life. I didn't know it at the time, but this lower-back pain was just a foreshadowing of the dreadful things to come. Within just a few short years, my health would rapidly spiral downward and almost completely out of control.

> This lower-back pain was just a foreshadowing of the dreadful things to come.

Even today, my recollection of the incident is almost perfect. I was in the backyard picking up some scrap wood and putting it into the garbage cart. As I was pulling the cart up to the house, I felt a razor-sharp pain in my lower back. I collapsed to the ground, immediately out of breath. *I have never felt this way before! Something is terribly wrong here.*

Playing basketball for decades had put a strain on my back, but this pain was something new and horribly different. I literally crawled to the house, got out an ice pack and promptly laid on it. The rest of the day and into the night was more of the same. Get up, get some ice, go over to the couch, and lay down again. The next morning, my back felt slightly better, but something else had occurred during the night. My sinuses were plugged up. *How strange!* I'd thrown my back out the day before, and now, the next morning, I was congested.

With the help of ice and ibuprofen, my back slowly got better. But the sinus congestion did not go away. So I did what millions of people do all around the world. I went to the local drugstore and bought a decongestant. From that point on, I used the decongestant daily. This went on for many months, and I went through a least a dozen bottles of various brands of decongestant before I sought professional help.

In the meantime, something else was happening to my body, and it was not for the better. One morning, my wife asked me what happened to my eye. *My eye? What's wrong with it?* I touched my face with my hand. My eye did feel strange. I went to the mirror and saw a puffy, discolored lump above and to the side of my eye. It looked like I had been punched. Well, I knew I hadn't been punched, but I thought that maybe I'd been bitten by a bug during the night. I have had black eyes in the past, and though this one looked like an eye that had been punched, it did not feel that way. It felt different, but I couldn't explain how or why.

More months passed, and though my back improved, my sinuses were a complete mess. I was constantly using a decongestant. I did this in spite of the fact that it appeared as if I was building up an immunity—some would say an addiction—to the decongestant. One squirt for the daytime and another before going to bed at night was no longer sufficient. Now I had to use the spray several times during the day and once or twice during the night. I didn't like what was happening to me, but I did not see a way out. I had no idea what was wrong. My sinuses were really becoming a problem. I talked to friends and got some advice for various cures, but nothing worked.

Ice and ibuprofen for the back. Decongestants for the sinuses. What I was doing was considered classic treatment in Western medicine. You have lower-back pain; you treat the lower back. You have clogged sinuses; you treat the clogged sinuses. Although attacking the problem where it is found seemed logical, in reality I was simply attacking the symptoms. I was not looking for underlying causes to the problems because frankly, I didn't think any underlying causes existed. Unfortunately, I didn't realize the faulty logic of addressing symptoms instead of causes until many years later. At this point in my journey, I simply did what I was told or what seemed logical to me. But attacking the symptoms provided only brief and temporary relief. My health problems did not improve. My body continued to deteriorate, and I spiraled downward.

CHAPTER 2

# Looking for Causes in All the Wrong Places

Despite my progressively worsening condition, I stubbornly held onto the notion that if I just took it easy for a while, all of these weird problems would go away. After all, this is how I had approached nearly all of my health problems previously, whether from sickness or injury. *Relax, Chris, don't push it. You really don't have to do anything now. Just take it easy for a while and you'll be better in no time. Before you know it, this will all be in the past.*

Well, I kept telling myself that for about a year and half, and it didn't do me any good at all. From the time I first threw out my back, I had witnessed a gradual decrease in overall wellness, and a slow but steady increase in weakness, confusion, apathy, frustration, and depression. During the eighteen months following that first incident with the garbage cart, I threw out my back several more times, used more decongestants than I care to recall, and swelled up frequently around the eyes, lips, and chin. All of this was happening for no apparent reason. On an almost regular basis, the swelling would occur at night while I was sleeping. Why did I wake up with the morning surprise of swelling so often? I had no answers. It was all so very strange and vexing.

I was a public-school science teacher at this time. Although I loved my job and my profession, my degrading health began to encroach on many things, including my career. I began to live my life on something of a day-to-day basis. I have a feeling people who have lived with chronic illness know exactly what this is like. If I swelled up during the night, I would assess my situation in the early morning hours and ask myself, "Am I fit for work today?" After a while, I think my students actually got used to me looking rather odd some mornings in class. And yes, every once in a while, a student would come up and say, "Uh, Mr. Dorais...what happened to your face?" At times the swelling and discoloration would be so bad that I would just call in sick for a day or two until it all subsided. It was embarrassing, inexplicable, and frustrating to be in such a state. But what was I to do?

Family and friends suggested I visit a chiropractor to get help for my back. I resisted this for quite a while because I was trying to fix my back the way I always had in the past, with ice and ibuprofen. But throwing my back out every few months was getting very old. As a matter of fact, I was beginning to act and feel very old. I was constantly on the ice, ibuprofen, and frequently flat on my back for sometimes days at a time. Finally, my frustration with a lower back that was in a total state of rebellion exceeded my stubbornly holding onto the idea that things would get better on their own, and I visited a local chiropractor for help.

My first visit to the chiropractor was both interesting and informative. The doctor was friendly and helpful. After a brief examination, he said that I was completely out of alignment, and I would have to come into his office two or three times a week for a while in order to get things corrected. I reluctantly agreed. We both knew that I had waited long enough—too long in fact—and nothing had changed for the better by the delay of treatment.

Over the next several months of chiropractic treatment, my back began feeling better. I found the treatments relaxing and even refreshing. The only aspect of the treatment that I did not like was the rapid twisting of my head. I imagined that the doctor, who was strong and weighed about 250 pounds, would someday twist so hard and fast that he would break my neck. But, keeping my imagination in check, I continued under the doctor's chiropractic care and seemed to receive some benefit from his work. However, even though I was now under chiropractic care, it seemed as if I was now throwing my back out more frequently than ever. Yes, the time needed to recover was shorter, but the frequency of these occurrences was greater. Perplexed with this, I tried a different chiropractor for a while, but nothing really changed. Although the chiropractic care was reducing my lower-back problems considerably, it was obvious to me that my overall health was not getting better. In fact, I seemed to be gradually getting worse. I wondered if my lack of improvement was because I needed to see yet another doctor, perhaps one who was more qualified to treat my condition. So I moved on and consulted with a third chiropractor and received some treatment from him. But after only a short period of time, I knew that wasn't working either.

I also asked the various doctors I had been seeing about the swelling and nasal issues I was having. None of these professionals had a definitive answer concerning these weird symptoms.

I continued on with chiropractic care until it seemed I was throwing out my back every few weeks. If you've ever done this, you understand the pain and frustration that accompanies it. The agony of a back that has been thrown out of alignment is almost unbearable. It is debilitating. So there I was—nasal problems, periodic facial swelling, and a lower back that refused to cooperate with professional treatment for any significant period of time. I was a disaster. Hunched over and feeling more miserable than ever, I started considering what was formerly unthinkable: lower-back surgery.

I consulted a friend of mine who had recently had surgery on his lower lumbar region. He'd had many of the same issues I was having, so I asked him for advice. His back was not in fantastic shape after the surgery, but he was mostly pain free. *Pain free*. This was exactly what I was after, a pain-free lower back. I consulted a few more people I knew who'd had back surgery. If surgery was indeed the next step for me, I wanted to be as prepared as possible before going under the knife. After speaking with many people concerning the benefits and drawbacks of surgery, I took my inquiries to the next level and consulted with a surgeon who was a back specialist. My visit with the specialist was brief. It consisted of some questions, and a quick physical inspection. It concluded with a very simple test.

"Try to touch your toes while bending down." I did this without too much difficulty. "Do you feel any pain when you are doing this?"

"No," I replied.

"You are probably not a good candidate for surgery—at least not yet." We then discussed his evaluation. He found that, while my back did show evidence of weakness, it was not to the level that actually warranted surgery. I was happy to hear this…sort of. I wanted to get better, and there I was, in an expert's office, paying a few hundred dollars for a twenty-minute consultation. My pursuit of good health was starting to add up in terms of cost, and I still wasn't getting closer to any real answers.

More time passed, and with the back problems continuing to aggravate me to no small degree, I decided to make an appointment with the prestigious University of Michigan Back and Pain Center. This world-class institution was located in my old college town. I had received two degrees from the University of Michigan, and I was hoping that Ann Arbor had one more gift for me, a pain-free back. It took some time just to get an appointment in the Back and Pain Center, but once the day finally came and I walked into the front lobby of the Center, I had a feeling this wasn't the place for me. I immediately felt humbled. All around me were people who were seriously disabled. The Back and Pain Center was teeming with men and women who were hunched over, barely able to walk at all. Wheelchairs, canes, and walkers were everywhere, and here I was, strolling in, looking for a quick fix so that I could get back to playing basketball. I may have been in bad shape, but I was a long way from looking like those poor folks. I left the Center with much of the same information I had received from the previous back specialist.

> I kept spending money seeing doctors, but always found myself back at square one.

"You are really not in that bad of shape, Mr. Dorais. If you can bend down and touch your toes fairly easily, this is not the place for you."

*Now what?* I wondered what my next move was going to be. I kept spending money seeing doctors, but always found myself back at square one. I was making no progress other than finding out what not to do. The "What Not to Do" list was getting longer while the "What to Do Next" list was nearly blank. I was tired, frustrated, and hurting.

Although I made no real progress on my back, I was starting to hear the word "allergy" more and more often when I spoke with people about my swelling. As far as I knew, I had never been allergic to anything in my life, but some people who saw me in my periodically swollen state said that it resembled an allergic reaction of sorts. So I started another crusade of looking to allergy specialists who might be able to make an accurate diagnosis and prescribe some sort of effective treatment. I suspected my symptoms were related because they all occurred at approximately the same time, but I did not know for sure. At this point, I just wanted healing. I wanted a respite from my health problems, and I wanted it now. Frankly, I was so very tired of seeing doctors and paying fees and getting no true, lasting relief. I needed answers, and these professionals were not giving them to me. My faith in the medical establishment and the doctors who were driving the system was slowly weakening. I still had faith in the system, but I was starting to have some doubts. This was not a good feeling. I felt the walls were closing in on me, and I had no idea what I was supposed to do or where I was going to turn to next.

# Chapter 3

# A New Level of Weird

I have known many people who have gone to see allergy specialists. I think it is safe to say that we have all heard stories of people who left the allergy clinic with a diagnosis that they were basically allergic to everything. Of course, many of these stories are pure fabrication or generous exaggeration, but I have to admit I had a preexisting skepticism regarding the accuracy of allergy tests. But I was desperate for answers, and because the word "allergy" seemed to creep up more and more in my search for answers, I decided to visit an allergy expert in the area. From all that I had heard and seen, this allergy doctor ran a thriving practice. He did not accept any insurance plans. After visiting his clinic only once, it was clear why he didn't accept insurance—he didn't need to. His clinic was packed with people, all of whom were willing to pay out-of-pocket costs in exchange for presumably excellent health-care services. I sat in the waiting room until it was finally my turn to be taken to an examination room.

Once inside an examination room, I waited again for the doctor. I already had some lab work done, and now it was time for a consultation with the doctor concerning the results. When the doctor came into the room, the first thing that I thought was how sick he looked! I realize this was a very bad first impression, and I hoped I was wrong with my instantaneous analysis, but I couldn't help it. The doctor appeared sickly, frail, and jaundiced. He was not at all what I was expecting. Although he seemed energetic, he also seemed a bit out of sorts. Frankly, I had a difficult time following his reasoning as he tried explaining his opinion of the lab results and his thoughts concerning my condition. At first I thought that perhaps it was just me. I wasn't able to follow his reasoning because he was just so much smarter than me. So I played the game. *You know, the game that you sometimes play with doctors.* Nod the head, smile thoughtfully, say yes frequently, and try to keep your mind from wandering as the good doctor rambles on and on. But my mind did wander. I thought less and less about what the doctor was saying, and more about how he was saying it. He seemed mechanical and rehearsed in his responses, almost as if he knew what he wanted to say to me without really looking at the data from my lab work. His "presentation," if that's what you want to call it, was scattered, disjointed, and vague. On top of this, again, he really did not seem to be in the best of health himself. My own observations notwithstanding, the doctor concluded that my existing lab work showed no obvious deficits, but it did point to a slight gluten allergy. He advised me to stay away from gluten in order to lower my allergic response. *Gluten allergy? That means wheat. But wheat has been around since Eden! Wow, I must really be in bad shape!*

> But wheat has been around since Eden! Wow, I must really be in bad shape!

He also recommended that I go on a rather extensive—and expensive—regimen of nutritional supplements. I was transfixed on his diagnosis and started thinking about how improbable it all sounded. My skepticism grew. As our consultation wrapped up, I learned that his office just coincidentally sold all of the expensive supplements he was recommending. *How convenient.*

Three hundred dollars for the consultation fee and another three to four hundred for supplements, all out-of-pocket. Not a bad sum of money for thirty minutes of the good doctor's time. I had no choice but to pay the consultation fee, but declined to purchase any of the supplements. Something just didn't seem right. It didn't add up. After paying the consultation fee in cash, I quickly left the office. I was angry and firmly convinced that I certainly would not be following any of the doctor's advice.

I had no plans to give up wheat—period. How was it possible for an adult to develop a food allergy to something as basic to the human diet as wheat? It just didn't make any sense at all. Eating bread had always been enjoyable for me, and I wasn't about to give it up, especially considering all of the circumstances surrounding the consultation with this "allergy specialist." In short, I thought the doctor was flat-out wrong. If gluten had really been the cause of my swelling, I think I would have determined that long before seeing him. I couldn't recall a single incident when I had eaten a generous portion of bread for dinner and the next morning had a swollen eye or lip.

But this office visit wasn't a complete waste. My bloodwork did show a slight sensitivity to gluten. Assuming the bloodwork was correct, this could be valuable information. People can, and often do, lie. But not numbers. Numbers can't lie. But they can be misinterpreted. I didn't think the doctor was lying, but I thought he was interpreting my data incorrectly. The bloodwork numbers were saying something, but I had no idea what. And I had a strong suspicion the doctor didn't know either. Something big was missing here, and I was certain it wasn't wheat, at least not directly. There must have been something behind the wheat, something deeper, but how this all linked to swelling, sinus problems, and backaches was a mystery. Even though this "something" was unknown to me at the time, clearly I needed to be even more diligent with what I ate. So that is exactly what I decided to do. If nothing unusual showed up after a few weeks, I would move on and look elsewhere for answers.

Well, it wasn't too long before things started to come a little more into focus. It had been about two years since the first time I'd thrown out my back. Through basic trial and error, I now finally started to see a possible connection between certain food types and my swelling. If I did swell up during the night (and it was almost always at night), it often occurred on days when I ate processed foods. But here is the weird thing—it didn't *always* happen with processed foods. My understanding of allergies at the time was that if you are allergic to Food X, you will have a reaction if you eat Food X.

In my case, Food X seemed to be a whole slew of different types of processed foods. Soups, crackers, cookies, snack chips, packaged meats, soft drinks—sometimes when I ate these foods, I would awake with a swollen eye or lip, and sometimes I would awake with no symptoms whatsoever. That was one of the most maddening things about my situation. I just could not replicate an allergic response on a consistent basis! And processed foods are everywhere. There were so many potential causes for this problem. I could not find a common denominator in any of this, but I did make one very important discovery. If I ate whole foods (fresh fruits, vegetables, meats) that had little or no processing, I was fine. I never reacted—ever—to eating a diet of pure, whole foods.

More time passed, and my frustrations mounted even as my overall health continued to decline. Because so many of my friends had mentioned allergies as a possible cause, and even though I had discussed my visit with the "no insurance allergy specialist" with many of them, I was persuaded to give allergy testing another try. I felt backed into a corner. I was a mess. My back was completely unpredictable, I was still swelling up regularly, and my sinuses were simply a disaster. And, there was more bad news on the horizon. I realized at this point that if it were possible to be truly and literally addicted to decongestants, then I was now a hard-core, bottle-sniffing junkie. I could no longer function without using a decongestant several times during the day and well into the night. I tried to limit my use of these typical all-purpose, over-the-counter decongestants. And I tried other homeopathic remedies, but the end result was still the same—congested sinuses. The bottom line was that I needed my decongestant because I simply could not breathe much of the time. Of course, this meant that sleeping was becoming a major problem. Before all of these health problems hit me, I had always begun my nights by sleeping on my stomach. I could no longer do this. My sinuses would plug up if I lay on my stomach, and I could not breathe out of my nose. Neither could I sleep on my back, as the same problem occurred. I found I could sleep by breathing through my mouth, but I would often awake in the middle of the night with an uncomfortably dry mouth and throat. Finally, after trying multiple sleeping positions, I found one that provided somewhat of a respite. For some unknown reason, I could breathe out of my nose if I went to sleep lying on my left side. I know this sounds strange, but it worked. So, sleeping on my left side began to be my nightly routine.

But, even as I found relief with my sleeping, another weird symptom started to occur. I began experiencing occasional swelling in and around my fingers and wrists. This swelling would also turn very itchy at times, and if I scratched to relieve the itch, the swelling would increase. *Sigh*. These weird symptoms were getting so very, very annoying. I had gone the chiropractor route, the back-specialist route, and the allergy-specialist route. I did not know where to turn next except to the allergy question again. I was still not convinced that allergies were at the root of my problems. It just didn't seem logical that a person could suddenly have sinus issues, lower-back pain, and periodic swelling because of some latent allergy problem. There seemed to be something bigger at play here, but again, I had no idea what it was.

I don't recall how I heard about this next place (so I have no person in mind right now to blame), but I found a clinic of allergy specialists who claimed to be able to rid a person of food allergies in a drug-free, noninvasive manner. This was exactly what I wanted. I also found that this allergy clinic accepted my insurance, so other than a thirty-dollar co-pay, the service was free. *Finally, I'd found someone who might be able to help me without further draining my bank account.*

After an initial consultation, I met with a therapist (not a doctor) who claimed to have cured numerous patients with a unique brand of healing. Intrigued, I asked what it was. She explained that many allergy cases like mine are actually psychological in nature, not physiological. Therefore, my psyche needed a sort of reprogramming and then a rebooting, so to speak. This would be done by—brace yourself for this—*speaking* to my body. Yes, you read that correctly. The therapist would *talk* my problems away. She said this with a completely straight face.

Since the sessions were covered by insurance and because the therapist was so optimistic that her treatments would work, I kept my weekly visits for about six weeks—which she said was the normal time for significant healing to occur. Well, perhaps to the surprise of absolutely no one but the therapist, I did not get better at all after six weeks of this farce. No healing. No change in me at all, except an ever-increasing level of skepticism for both traditional and nontraditional medical treatments. On my very last visit to the office of this allergy specialist, I gently confronted the therapist and reminded her of what she'd told me six weeks earlier about how successful these sessions were for other patients. She seemed rather surprised at this and like a magician whose magic act doesn't work on stage, she rather awkwardly made up some reason or another as to why I needed to come back for more extensive sessions.

"If you come back for more *blah blah blah*, you should finally see some progress in your condition," she unblinkingly stated.

I thanked her for her time and said I would consider it. But by the time I had reached the exit door, I had decided this was all quite ridiculous and I was never coming back. Angry for being taken in by this not-so-slick snake-oil saleswoman, I resolved to be far more diligent and disciplined in my research, so as not to ever fall for a trap like this one again. Alas, it would be only a few months later that I would be duped once more, and this next mistake was ridiculously costly.

# Chapter 4

# Please Pass the Snake Oil

More time passed, and my health continued its gradual downward trajectory. I hadn't gotten much help from the allergy experts that I had consulted, but I did listen to some of their advice concerning my diet. I had always eaten pretty much whatever I wanted to eat, but now it seemed as if those days were gone forever. I was paying much closer attention to what I was eating, but still I would awake with that awful swelling from time to time. And things were getting worse. Not only was I experiencing swelling on my fingers, wrists, eyes, and mouth, but occasionally I would awaken in the morning with hives, usually on my back or buttocks. These hives were red, itchy, lumpy, and would typically last for six to twelve hours. I could not figure out what was causing them. The hives and swellings still seemed to be related to certain processed foods, but I couldn't consistently demonstrate what the offending cause or causes were. The unpredictability of these allergic reactions was maddening. There was very little, if any, consistency to my allergic reactions, if that was what they were.

> *The unpredictability of these allergic reactions was maddening.*

I don't actually recall when or where it happened, but at some very low point, I decided to give those nutritional supplements another look—you know, the ones that I was advised to take after my first allergy test. Actually I was going to give it more than just another look. My health and future were more important than money, so I decided to go full-throttle into the realm of nutritional supplements. I resolved to spare no expense in my search for answers, even with the priciest of supplements. And while I was at it, I figured I might as well try some of the less traditionally known treatments for back inflammation, too. I was so low, and in so much pain, that this new resolve was more of an act of desperation and a cry for help than a logical decision. But my back was giving me major problems. At times, it seemed as if it were on fire. The pain was not chronic yet, but it seemed to be approaching that threshold very rapidly.

Along with buying a plethora of expensive vitamin and nutritional supplements, I spent a considerable amount of money on quick and often unusual health remedies. One such foray into the exotic was my purchase of a mattress pad loaded with high-powered magnets. This pad promised to be an amazing cure for all matters related to an aching back. I can laugh at this now, but only until I remember its rather substantial price tag. I used this magnetic mattress for several months. But after a while, with no improvement evidenced at all, I concluded either my problems were too severe for this mattress to solve or magnetic medicine of this sort was a sham. In any event, I did eventually find one excellent use for the mattress. It might not have done anything good for my aching back, but I was quite comfortable lying on it while draining the oil from my truck's oil pan.

About this time, I started reading a book about a man who was suffering from Crohn's disease. According to the book, the man had literally become an eighty-pound weakling who had tried a variety of different treatments in the hope of finding a cure for this horrible intestinal disease. If you do not know anything about Crohn's disease, I suggest you do a bit of research on it. My mother had suffered from Crohn's before she passed away, so many of this author's stories personally resonated with me. The bottom line to the book was that people who have digestive issues (and I assumed that was me), need to radically change their diet. This included a drastic reduction in junk foods, highly processed foods, and much, if not most, restaurant food.

The overall recommendation of the book was to eat whole foods, and to avoid foods that contained a great deal of manmade additives. The author claimed that, over the course of a year or two, he had been able to beat Crohn's disease and recover his health through this new diet and a generous inclusion of nutritional supplements.

Now wouldn't you know it, but these same supplements were conveniently offered by this author's newly formed nutritional company. And of course, the supplements were very pricey. If this whole story sounds a bit familiar—and it should—it's because I'd been down this road before.

You may be thinking at this point that I was an insanely naïve and desperate person to fall for this old snake oil trap again. Maybe I was, but there was a simple reason for it all. *I was desperate.* True desperation has few boundaries, particularly when it comes to health and money. But even in this state of desperation, I was trying to analyze this situation as objectively as I could. Getting away from junk food was something I had been trying to do for some time. I did not see any connection between the junk food I ate and my lower-back pain, but there did sometimes seem to be a connection between the junk food and the swelling and hives. I still couldn't find any consistent food or chemical trigger, but I was not yet really taking the reading of food labels seriously. This is kind of sad and slightly pathetic, because I was a high school chemistry teacher at the time. *Sigh.* I seem to have left all my chemistry-related knowledge and experience at the schoolhouse. It didn't make it to my own house in those early years, and that obviously was a big mistake.

In any event, I decided that maybe there was some usefulness in the nutritional supplements mentioned in the book, so I started buying and taking them. This went on for some time. And, even though I was somewhat jaded by the whole "nutritional supplement syndrome," as I called it, I began to add more and more supplements to my diet. I kept thinking that maybe the answer was just around the corner. I kept telling myself that there had to be some truth to the claims that the nutritional supplement companies made concerning their products. *They couldn't stay in business long if their products didn't provide some benefit...right?* I was spending larger and larger sums of money on pills, in the hope that they would bring the relief I was looking for. I just had to get my health back.

Before judging my naïveté too harshly, please consider the desperate nature of my circumstances. In a very short span of time, my freedom to enjoy foods that I had eaten for years was nearly gone. To make matters worse, this freedom and joy of eating was replaced by a nebulous enemy I couldn't even identify. Sometimes foods would cause painful and embarrassing allergic reactions, and sometimes these same foods would not cause any problems at all. Maybe this is what bothered me the most. I could not predict anything, and so I ate in a state of fear. It wasn't so much about food, as it was about freedom, and the sudden loss of it. Without freedom, all that is left is a prison—a cage. That is how I felt now. This was my bitter new reality.

CHAPTER 5

# A Slight Paradigm Shift

They say that necessity is the mother of invention. This may be true for many people, but for me, it was more desperation that was the mother of invention. I had been fighting this declining health syndrome for well over two years now and, sadly, I really didn't have many answers. In fact, I really had no answer except that, up to this point, just about everything I was doing to improve my health was wrong. In one sense, I suppose this was a good thing. At least I knew what not to do. I also had enough courage to admit that I was an abject failure as a self-healer.

Once you hit rock bottom, the only place left to go to is up, right? Hitting the bottom caused a paradigm shift of sorts in my overall strategy. I began to look at things from a different perspective. I still had no idea what was wrong with me in terms of particulars, but as I looked at my situation in more generalized terms, a few things started to come into focus.

My problems seemed to have something to do with nutrition and manmade substances. How had I come to this conclusion? Well, I was weak—weaker than I had ever been before. My back was a complete mess and an almost constant source of pain and irritation. I was having trouble with my memory. Physically and mentally, it seemed that I was aging at a wildly accelerated rate. I just felt so very old and fragile. If someone were to tell me all of these symptoms, I would have thought that they were not eating the right foods. But I was eating the right foods now, and I was taking a huge amount of expensive nutritional supplements to make up for whatever was lacking in my diet. But all of this eating of the right foods and taking nutritional supplements did not halt my health decline. It seemed as if I wasn't getting the benefits that I needed from the foods that I had been eating. So I reasoned that I must have some sort of nutritional deficiency that was caused, not by inferior food *consumption*, but by inferior food *absorption*.

The other side of my problems were the allergic reactions. When I ate whole foods, I had no trouble with swelling or hives. Sometimes—and still only sometimes—when I ate processed foods (and I define "processed" as anything that contains chemical additives), I would swell up and/or get hives. But I had been eating processed foods my whole life, and nothing like this had happened before. This told me that, for some unknown reason, I now had a powerful chemical *sensitivity*. I was fairly certain my back problems were somehow related to a nutritional deficiency and chemical sensitivity, but exactly how it was related was totally beyond me.

With all of this in mind, I decided to take it very easy on my back, ice it constantly, and really focus my energies on what I thought were my two main problems—a nutritional deficiency and a chemical sensitivity.

I have heard people say "you have to listen to your body." Honestly, that had always sounded kind of crazy to me...until now. I began to take daily note of what my body was doing, how it looked, and how I felt. Yes, by this point in my journey, I really was trying to listen to my body. And what did my body say to me? Well, as strange as this sounds, I thought my body was telling me it was slowly being poisoned.

> ...I thought my body was telling me it was slowly being poisoned.

As a science teacher, I felt I had a fairly comprehensive understanding of how the body works. I also thought I had an ample understanding of the biochemistry involved. Looking back years later, I realize that this was not true at all. Actually, at this point in my journey, I had only a rudimentary understanding of the biochemistry at work within me. Despite my ignorance, I was moving forward. If I was reading the signals correctly that I was, in fact, being slowly poisoned, I needed to know both why and how it was happening. To do this, I would have to take my science understanding out from the theoretical sense of a classroom and put it to good practical use with my own body. But there was a problem. All of my training and education was theoretical and objective. It was designed to test and experiment "out there," not "in here." My education and training was for the science laboratory—in a room, in a building; not in a body. And especially not in my body. This was a big shift, because it would require me to personally test my own theories. But to do actual experiments on myself was not something that I wanted to do. I wanted the experts to tell me what to do. I wanted doctors to give me an accurate diagnosis and a workable treatment plan.

You know the routine. Listen to your doctors, do what they say, take all of the medications they prescribe, and sooner or later…you're better. But I had tried to do this for the last couple of years, and it hadn't worked out. I was looking around for other options, but there just weren't any that I hadn't already tried. I was on my own.

What I needed to do now was to treat my own condition as one of my classroom experiments. If what I was eating was causing me some problems, then I would document both the food and the problems. I would also have to become quite proficient in reading and understanding food label ingredients. Maybe I could isolate one of these ingredients as being the cause of my problems.

In short, I decided to go back to the basics—to do research, collect data, and test theories. All of this would be necessary so that I could experiment…on myself. This new paradigm shift was sort of like going back to school in a way. I would have to become much more proficient in doing both research and experimentation. Scholarly studies, government publications, books, articles, websites, blogs—I would need to gather data from all of these sources. Also, I would be paying much closer attention to the little clues my body gave me on a daily basis as to its operation and function.

I understood the science information that came from a textbook. But gaining an understanding as to why my own body's systems were failing to respond to the various protocols I had already used was a completely different matter. My body was failing on a biochemical level, and I needed to know why. I didn't know much at this point—almost nothing really—so actually, this was a great place to start.

There is hope when ignorance is coupled with humility. At least you know you don't know anything, and you are willing to listen and learn because you are humble about it. But if ignorance is coupled with arrogance, look out. There is little hope for that person, until of course, they hit rock bottom. And that was me. I had hit rock bottom. I was ready to go back to school.

It was now approximately two and a half years since that first incident of pulling the garbage cart in my backyard. While I am not exactly sure of the total amount of money I had spent so far, I estimate it to be about $25,000. Sadly, I didn't have much to show for this money. I had a cupboard full of supplements, none of which seemed to help me at all. I had a magnetic mattress that doubled as an oil drop cloth on my garage floor. I had a body that was in complete rebellion, and I had very few answers going forward.

Even as my paradigm shift gave me new hope and perspective, my health continued to plummet. New health issues were cropping up. One of the more strange problems that now presented itself was with my feet. I was taking a shower one day, and suddenly I felt a shooting pain in my foot. My initial thought was that I had stepped on something. I looked for some sharp object on the shower floor, but there was nothing there. I just felt this pain. Then, slowly the pain turned to a sort of aching and moved its way to the top of my foot. It's difficult to describe really—not a pain in the joints, but rather in and around the tendons. It felt like thousands of tiny pins were poking the top of my foot. It was terribly painful. I began stamping my foot down, thinking that for some reason my foot had fallen asleep. But feet don't typically fall asleep while one is standing in the shower. Later that day, as I was walking around, it began to feel as if there was something in my shoe. It actually felt as if there was an extra sole on the bottom of my foot. I took a closer look, and I found what was wrong. The sole of my foot was swollen. *What is happening to me? I am just falling apart and I have no idea why!*

My first thought was that perhaps this was a result of the many supplements I was taking. But then I began to suspect that the supplements might actually heal the foot problem. Yes, I am sure you are thinking that I was going around in circles with my reasoning. You are right. I was chasing my tail, but at the time I saw no other choice. Doing nothing was not an option. I had already tried that door, and my problems had only gotten worse. I could not sit around and wait for things to improve. I had to do something.

I got back into the research. I began to think that perhaps I was missing a key vitamin, mineral, or enzyme in my diet. If I could just find that missing ingredient, my health would improve. So I took the plunge and purchased even more bottles of vitamins, minerals, food enzymes, essential oils, and other supplements. I even ordered a few packs of those detox foot patches that were advertised on late-night cable TV shows. Manufacturers of the patches proposed that the body is full of toxins, and one of the avenues through which the body eliminates toxins is sweat. Since our feet sweat, we place these special patches on our feet, and the chemicals in them would draw the toxins out of the body and into the patches. This was to be done typically at night. In the morning, the patches would be discolored and malodorous, due to the toxins that had been drawn out of the body.

Well, I did see a basic working logic with these so-called detox foot patches. I was especially motivated to use something on my feet, because of the swelling and arthritic pain I was having there. Honestly, I wasn't sure what true arthritis felt like, and while I thought I was far too young to have arthritis, my symptoms were similar to those who did have it. I stuck with the foot patches for several months in the hope of finding some measure of relief.

More time passed and even more money was spent before I was finally convinced that those foot patches and all of the supplements I had been taking were doing me little, if any, good at all. I had been using the foot patches and taking huge doses of supplements for several months, and I still had every single annoying symptom that I had before I started this regimen. All of my previous problems were still present and accounted for, and sadly, more weird and irritating symptoms seemed just over the horizon. I asked myself some brutally honest questions about what I had been doing the last few years, and wondered if it had all been a big waste of time and money. *Were all of the doctors I had consulted with simply quacks practicing junk medicine? Were all those supplements I had been taking just old-fashioned snake oil?*

I wasn't sure one way or the other. Most of these doctors and so-called health experts seemed like honest, hard-working professionals. I have no doubt that many of their products and services can and do help many people. Their business would not survive for long if it were otherwise. But I did not receive the help that I needed. As selfish as this may sound, I was primarily interested in results for me, not the good intentions of these health professionals. All I was sure of at this point was that I was now about three years into my journey, and I had spent approximately $35,000 out-of-pocket.

Despite the fact that my symptoms continued to worsen, my new focus on research did produce some valuable first fruits. I was beginning to see commonalities between my various ailments, my own personal research, the experiences that I'd had, and what I had been hearing from the many people I had consulted for medical advice. These commonalities became the basis for what I called my "Theory of Everything." This theory had four elements that guided my thinking process as I moved forward with my investigation. The four elements of the theory were as follows:

1. **The answer I was looking for was probably a combination of things, because my health dilemma was most likely a combination of problems.** As I have already mentioned, it took about three years and somewhere around $35,000 to figure this out. This dollar amount is a very rough estimate, because I frequently ignored looking at the receipts for doctor bills and nutritional supplements. I deliberately did some rather sloppy accounting on how much I was actually spending, because frankly, the real

numbers just became too depressing. However, as I stepped back and began looking at my situation with some real perspective, an idea began to solidify in my mind. There was not just one single ailment, toxin, parasite, virus, or whatever at play here. Surely I was dealing with a multifaceted problem, because so many different things were going wrong with my body. Since the problem was multifaceted, it seemed reasonable to assume the solution must also be multifaceted.

2. **The answer for my health problems *did* exist, and I was determined to find it. But, my solution had to be cost effective, easy to understand, easy to do, and fairly quick in its operation.** Obviously at this point in my journey, I had far more questions than answers. To be completely candid, I really didn't even know what most of the questions should be. But I believed my sickness was happening for a reason, and I knew one of the reasons was that, once the answers were found, I could share them with other people who were suffering just as I was. I knew there were answers out there that could bring my health back. But I wanted more than just an answer to my health problems. I wanted to find a solution that was elegantly simple, reasonably priced, and would show results fairly quickly. I had been searching for answers for three years now. If the healing protocol did not have the elements of simplicity, cost-effectiveness, and efficiency, most people (including myself) simply would not do it. I had faith a protocol for my health problems existed—I just had to find it.

3. **The problem was not *out there* but *in here*.** There is a big difference between chasing causes and chasing symptoms. I was fairly certain at this point that although outside factors like food seemed to be aggravating my condition and eliciting an allergic response, my real problems had to be internal. The issues with my back and the swelling and hives were not due to something that I was currently doing, nor were they from something I'd had a one-time exposure to. I had not made any drastic changes in my

lifestyle that would bring on my unknown sickness. My problem had already been inside of me. Inside of me was where I needed to effect changes first. This is why all those supplements did me very little good. There was something already drastically wrong with me on the inside that was far beyond the reach of any outside supplement to fix. What exactly this was—I had no idea. But if my problems could have been solved by supplements, it would have already happened by now.

4. **The problem in me had something to do with the element** *sulfur*. I know this may sound very random to you. It did to me too. *Sulfur? Why sulfur?* Over the course of the last few years, sulfur just seemed to keep popping up on my radar. I'm a chemistry guy. I love the subject. So when I kept hearing things concerning sulfur deficiency or issues with the sulfur-hydrogen bonds in proteins or the sulfur connection with detoxification, I finally began to pay attention. Call it a hunch if you like, but sulfur came up so many times in my budding investigation that I decided it was just too important to ignore. Intuitively, I felt sulfur was somehow a key player in the mystery illness I was dealing with, but how exactly it fit into the puzzle was unknown at the time.

As a teacher and student of the sciences, I am a huge fan of the Occam's razor. In its most basic form, Occam's razor states that nature takes the path of least resistance. I envision the razor as nature's toolbox for accomplishing work. This work could be either helpful or harmful to people. So, as it applied to my body, some very simple things had gone wrong with me, and I got sick. But if simple things were the cause of my illness, then simple things could also be the cause for my cure. There are people everywhere who were just like me, suffering from sickness unknown, and looking for answers. It did not seem logical that all of those people would have problems stemming from different sources. Rather, it seemed logical that people like me were sick because of very similar sources—or even one single source. If this assumption was correct, then logically the answer would also be in agreement with Occam's razor. The answer would be relatively uncomplicated.

I was not saying that the underlying biochemistry involved was not complicated. On the contrary, I was sure that the biochemistry involved was quite complex. But the beauty of this thought was that I didn't really have to understand it all. I didn't even have to understand most of it. I just needed to understand a few of the most critical, key pieces of the puzzle.

Call it pure intuition, but I also felt that, even though the biochemical mechanisms were incredibly complex, finding a cure that was basic in terms of the raw materials required and how these were related was probably relatively simple. I didn't need to find some rare species of flower growing only in the Amazonian rainforest for my cure. If Occam's razor was working to destroy my health, it stood to reason that this same razor could be used to bring healing as well. In fact, the answers should be fairly easy to find. They might even be hiding in plain sight.

As it turns out, many of the answers were, in fact, hiding in plain sight. And I would later discover that I was at least partially right on all four elements of my Theory of Everything. But it would take nearly nine more years of exploration, and an astonishing number of failures before I would finally discover these answers.

CHAPTER 6

# Asking the Right Questions

More time passed, and my problems continued to increase in severity. The lower-back pain was not constant, but it was very bothersome, and when it did flare up, it was pure agony. I was still under chiropractic care, and while this provided temporary relief, it was usually short-lived. At this point, the swelling and hives were my greatest concerns. I was experiencing an almost daily occurrence of swelling around the eye, lip, foot, or fingers. The hives were becoming more severe as well. Those red patches of skin were now larger than ever, itchy, and very uncomfortable. I was extremely cautious with what I was eating, and yet I was still having these all-too-regular outbreaks. In fact, the swellings and hives were happening so often with so many different types of foods, I was beginning to become apathetic to it all. *What is the use of paying such close attention to my diet if I still swell up all of the time anyway?*

Settled into a complacent apathy was not where I wanted to be, nor was it really in my nature. But after more than three years of seeing my symptoms progressively worsen, I had a very difficult time keeping an optimistic attitude in all of this. I needed a breakthrough of some sort, even if it was only a very small one. I needed something to give me a little hope.

Well, at just the right time, I found a glimmer of that hope. I had known for some time that I seemed to do extremely well when I ate only whole foods—fresh fruits, meats, grains, and vegetables. *This has to mean something! But what's causing me problems—the chemical additives in processed foods?* Unfortunately, while I knew that eating whole foods provided a huge amount of relief from the hives and swelling, I also found that eating whole foods exclusively was not at all convenient to my preferred lifestyle. The allure of my old eating habits was often stronger than my aversion to the hives and swelling, and I sometimes rebelled against the all-whole-foods diet that had been proven so many times to be safe for me. Far too frequently, I shamefully confess, I would take chances with food—particularly restaurant food. Why? Convenience, habit, apathy, and laziness are probably the best four reasons for this. But, as any risk-taker knows, sooner or later it catches up with you. It always does. It caught up with me in a big way while I was on vacation in Washington D.C.

We were taking a short family vacation in the nation's capital. In terms of food, there was not too much to choose from that could really be considered whole foods, but I tried to make the best of it. I was eating out for every meal. For anyone with food allergy issues, eating out can be a bit of a challenge. After just one day of eating like this, I started to feel a little sick. But we were doing so much walking and sightseeing, I tried not to focus too much on how I felt. By the last day of the trip, however, it caught up with me. My face felt itchy all over, particularly in my chin area. So, like anyone else, I scratched and rubbed my chin until I felt a measure of relief. By the time I got home from Washington, my chin was so completely swollen that I looked almost cartoonish. My chin was absolutely huge; it was swelling on a whole new level. In spite of the severity of the swelling, I treated this episode like any other. I simply ignored it. It's what I had always done in the past, and the swelling usually subsided after a few hours.

Later that evening, I was invited to a friend's house for a cookout. My chin still looked ridiculously large, but the swelling had decreased somewhat. And of course, when I showed up, my friends made jokes about how my "cartoon chin" was the latest and greatest physical oddity they had seen on me yet. They were, sadly, quite used to seeing me look rather strange at times, as was I. In any event, on the menu for dinner that night was just what you might expect with a bunch of guys cooking out—pure junk food. We ate hot dogs and chips, drank soda, and passed the evening with stories and laughter.

By the next morning, I wasn't laughing anymore.

I awoke feeling a tightness and heaviness all over my face. My wife looked at me with shock and pleaded in desperation that I stop playing doctor and go see another specialist. I went to the mirror and saw two grossly swollen lips, and both of my cheeks were puffy and swollen as well. I looked so horrible it was actually scary.

I had eaten at so many different locations in Washington that I really didn't know where to start. But I knew exactly what I had eaten at the cookout. I started thinking about the Washington food and the cookout food, and I made an assumption. *My chin began to swell while I was still in Washington, and now I have swelling all over my face. I must have eaten the same problem food twice.* I was on to something. Even though I was miserable, I was motivated by the clues that were staring me in the face.

Actually, looking back, I can see a huge number of clues that I completely missed over the years. But I was glad that at least now I was on to something that really had the potential to provide some much-needed answers. I focused my attention on the processed foods I had eaten at the cookout: hot dogs, buns, chips, soda, ketchup, mustard. But the ingredients on the labels of these foods didn't mean anything to me—at least not yet. I needed help in making sense of what was on these labels. Then I had an idea.

> I needed help in making sense of what was on these labels. Then I had an idea.

I had already consulted several allergy experts in the medical field and had gotten almost nowhere. It was now time to take my investigation to another level—to the experts in the *field of life*. I am referring here to the many mothers who have children with food allergies. I began talking to moms to learn what they knew about food allergies. Over and over, the term "monosodium glutamate" (MSG) kept popping up in our conversations. *Very interesting.* These moms asked if I had considered MSG as a potential allergen. I said that I had not. I wasn't even sure I knew what MSG was.

Like so many people, I thought MSG was a chemical used in cheap restaurants. But considering everything that I had already gone through, the idea of MSG being a causal agent of at least some of my symptoms seemed quite possible. I did a little research on monosodium glutamate, and it turned out that the standard MSG allergic reaction did seem to match many of my own symptoms. *Whoa...this was a surprise.* I went back and examined some of the labels of the foods that I had eaten at the cookout. Sure enough, there it was, right on the label of the bag of chips: monosodium glutamate. MSG was in my absolute favorite snack. *Ouch.* I loved those chips. I had been eating them my whole life. I'd had no idea that they contained MSG, but in all honesty, even if I had known it, I doubt if I would have cared. Let's be honest—few people read the labels of the foods they eat, because very few people really care about what is in their food. And even if they did care, would they understand the significance or the effects of the many chemicals in their foods? I doubt it. So here I was, wondering what MSG was and what it did to me, and I was a chemistry teacher. *Ouch again.*

Well, now I really started paying attention to food labels; I read them all the time—and everywhere. Surprisingly, I found that MSG did not show up too frequently on food labels. Yes, I did find it in some foods on the store shelf, but it wasn't on the label as much as I thought it would be. In fact, there were several foods that I thought were possible causes of my swellings and hives, but MSG wasn't on their labels. This was weird. I didn't expect this. Gradually I began to discover that my new theory regarding a potential MSG allergy wasn't even close to being consistent with what I had experienced.

In any event, after all of my talks with the moms and all of the food label reading, and after doing a small amount of research on MSG, I decided it was time to do an experiment. I wanted to test my so-called MSG Allergy Theory, and the only way to do this was to potentially cause myself some discomfort. So I sat down one evening and purposely ate food that had the words "monosodium glutamate" listed right on the food label. Sure enough, about seven hours later, my face and lips began tingling and getting itchy, and about two hours after that, I had two fat and swollen lips.

Even though this was a painful experiment, I was happy that I had made my first real discovery.

I officially self-diagnosed myself as being allergic to MSG.

Of course, at this juncture, I had no idea *why* I was allergic to MSG. I also did not know why this apparent allergy had come on so suddenly just a few years ago, when I had been eating food with MSG my whole life. I couldn't remember any swelling incidents before that time. But something was different with my body, beginning that day when I was in my backyard pulling that garbage cart with the scrap wood. What this difference was I had no idea, but I knew it wasn't good. The positive in all of this was that now I had MSG in my sights, and it was something I could clearly avoid when buying food.

But it wasn't that easy. Old habits die hard, and I had a habit of eating out fairly regularly. Reading labels before buying food and eating it is one thing, but eating food at a restaurant is something else entirely. How could I know whether or not the restaurant used MSG in their foods? At first I tried asking the cooks, waiters, and waitresses about MSG. Very few ever said, "Oh yes, we put MSG in many of our foods!" I was new to all of this, and I thought I was just asking an honest question. *You see, at this point I had not yet learned the rules of the game.* I found out later that, almost without exception, no one in the food business wants to admit that they put MSG in their products. In addition to this, I honestly believe very few restaurant workers even know what is in their foods. They were just like me—blissfully ignorant of all those strange-sounding chemicals listed on the food label.

I was at a crossroads with this MSG situation, because I loved eating out. For a while, I just took my chances. I decided I would eat out, but only at places that *looked clean*. But this plan didn't work. I quickly found that I would swell up from food from several different places, many of which were very popular, big-name restaurants. Trial and error just seemed like such a painful way to proceed along this path.

Was there a better way to guard against MSG? I wasn't sure. In fact, what did I even know about MSG? Not much, really. In the small amount of research that I had done, I'd found that MSG symptoms closely matched my own. I also found that MSG is used in foods as a flavor enhancer. Frankly, I thought that MSG was probably harmless to most people. *After all, companies wouldn't deliberately put things in our food that could actually harm us...right?* Looking back now, I see how blithely naïve I was about this whole thing. With so many more questions than answers on the subject, I decided to really dig into the research on monosodium glutamate.

Here is the basic molecular structure of MSG. I found in my research that MSG is a chemical added to foods to mask a portion of the food that tastes bitter or unpleasant. MSG does not really have a flavor of its own. Instead, it has a rather unique ability to enhance the brain's perception of the existing flavor of the food that it is mixed into. *Very clever.* But I found more, much more, about this curious substance.

When people defend MSG as being "all natural," I suppose this is true in a literal sense, but not really in the sense that most people understand. Yes, MSG can be derived from all natural sources, so in this sense it truly is "all natural." But this is a word game that food manufacturers play. The MSG that is added to our food is done so at a far higher concentration than anything that is found in nature. Ultra-high concentrations of this chemical are sprayed onto foods in order to give them a decidedly unnatural natural flavor. Do some research on why MSG is called an "excitotoxin" and you may see what I mean.

Many weeks passed, and I was dutifully reading my food labels in order to steer clear of MSG. I began seeing progress, swelling up less frequently after meals. As some of you already know, living with a food allergy can be dreadful, but it is far better to be living with a known allergy than an unknown one. Although I had isolated MSG as an offending chemical and was trying very hard to avoid it, I *still* experienced that irritating swelling from time to time. Even when the labels didn't mention MSG, certain foods caused an allergic reaction. When I say "certain foods," I am referring mostly to processed ones—which, of course, are foods that come in a package, bottle, or can. Typically, processed foods have lengthy lists of added chemicals, and this, I learned, is where things get tricky.

Why did certain foods that did not contain MSG instigate an allergic reaction? And why did this allergic reaction occur only sometimes? There was still so much that I did not know, but I was working on it. By now I was reading labels very diligently, but certain processed foods—particularly canned soups—still caused an allergic response. It seemed that I must also be allergic to chemicals other than MSG. But finding what those chemicals might be was extremely difficult.

I decided that it was time to conduct another experiment. Since I needed to control every aspect of my eating, I first made the decision to forego eating at any restaurant for a few weeks. There were simply too many variables to control at a restaurant. Next, I would eat only whole foods for a time, and then slowly add in certain processed foods, carefully noting what was on each food label. With the successful MSG discovery now behind me, I had a new motivation in my quest. It seemed as if I was finally starting to ask the right questions, and I was determined to find more answers with this experiment. I began my experiment using a highly controlled diet, and it didn't take too long once I started adding in processed foods again before I swelled up. Thankfully, the swelling was not as severe as it had been in the past, but I had a nice reddish and puffy eye from something I ate. I went back and reviewed the labels of the foods that I had eaten over the last twelve hours. Not much attracted my attention, except that some of the foods contained an ingredient called "natural flavors." *Natural flavors? Hmm. Sounds harmless enough...even healthy!*

I brushed off my suspicions about "natural flavors," whatever they were. I thought maybe I had missed something else along the way, something important. So I went on with my experiment. A short while later, I had another allergic reaction. I went back and looked over all of the labels again. *This is weird. Nothing seems out of place here...calcium carbonate, potassium nitrate, natural flavors. Hmm. There it is again: natural flavors.*

I went to the pantry and began reading the labels of every food product that was there. I was shocked at how many times "natural flavors" showed up on the label. I had not noticed this before. But there it was, right before me, hidden in plain sight. Even my favorite chocolate cookies had "natural flavors" on the label. This was bad. I was already having a tough time changing my eating habits, and this discovery had just made my lifestyle adjustment even harder. Whatever these "natural flavors" actually contained was a complete mystery, but it certainly appeared as if they were a villain. But how could MSG or "natural flavors" affect my back? The swelling and rashes had begun within days of that initial episode with my back, when all of my health problems first started. I felt certain the two were related. But how? I still had no idea.

And my bad back was giving me major problems. If you have never had lower-back pain, consider yourself fortunate. The best word that comes to mind—and I used it quite often in those days—is *debilitating*. Lower-back pain is a terribly debilitating condition. It affects everything you do. You sit in pain. You walk gingerly because of the pain. You say no to normal activities because of the pain. You consciously avoid even simple movements that most people do, because you think you might end up hurting your back. In short, normal life becomes a pain.

One day I was sitting at my desk, and I dropped my pencil. With my legs under the desk and the pencil on the ground to the side of me, I twisted my trunk as I bent down to pick up the pencil. *Ping....there went my lower back.* It was that easy. Needless to say, I was in a very fragile state when something as simple as picking up a pencil could cause such agonizing pain. I usually found that after several days of rehabilitating myself, a visit or two to the chiropractor, and plenty of ice, I would be back to my normal, abnormal self.

My back issues had actually become quite a conversation piece with friends and acquaintances. "Hey Chris, how is that back of yours?" In case you are wondering, having a bad back as a conversation piece is not a good thing. I don't recall now who actually gave me the idea, but it came to my attention that there were some fairly inexpensive nutritional supplements that could be taken for lower-back pain. *Inexpensive supplements that had a good track record of reducing back pain?* I was all in.

From the information that I'd received from my many doctors, friends, and my own personal research, I'd found that chronic lower-back problems were typically characterized as being in a state of constant inflammation. If I could find a way to reduce that inflammation, I might see some reduction in pain. It sounded like a reasonable theory, and trying a few more supplements was definitely a welcome alternative to surgery.

One such supplement that got my attention was called *methylsulfonylmethane*, or MSM. (Yes, that word is a mouthful—what were those chemists thinking?!) When I read about MSM and its claims as an all-natural anti-inflammatory supplement, I was interested, but skeptical. After my previous research with food labels, I was fairly suspicious with any claim that something was "all natural." MSG also claimed to be all natural, and I knew what that stuff did to me. I wondered if MSM would be any different. I started slowly with a minimal dosage, and the first thing I noticed was that it did not cause any allergic swelling. That was a good thing. *First, do no harm...right?* I gradually took larger doses until I found a level where MSM did make a significant difference with my lower-back pain. I also found that MSM also gave a much-needed boost to my overall energy, which was pretty pathetic in those days. I did a little research and found that methylsulfonylmethane is produced by the cells of the human body for a variety of reasons, not the least of which was the reduction of inflammation. It certainly worked for me. The MSM seemed to douse much of the pain in my lower back, which oftentimes felt like it was on fire. The only real concern was the quantity of MSM I needed to take in order to see a real decrease in the level of pain. I had worked my way up to about twenty 500 mg pills of MSM daily. This is 10 grams of MSM. That was the amount I needed before I felt the abatement of pain. From all I could find in the research, MSM is nontoxic at that amount, so I felt confident going forward that I was not contributing to my problems. I did not like the idea of having to take so many pills to get relief, but I was desperate, and the MSM did provide a significant measure of pain reduction.

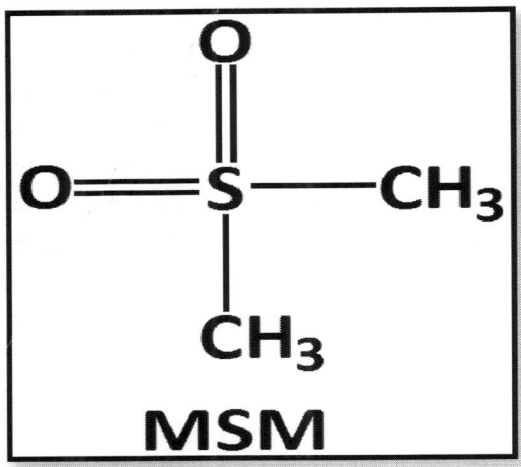

I was so happy about my MSM discovery that I dug into the research even more on this fascinating substance. In addition to its anti-inflammatory capabilities, MSM has the ability to repair soft tissue, like cartilage. This was really good news, because I had been wondering if I had damaged the disks of my lower back from the many times I had thrown it out. I had imagined my lower discs were in pretty bad shape, and since discs are made of cartilage, I was hoping that my back would begin to heal as a result of taking MSM. Also—and this was the really interesting part—MSM contained the element *sulfur*! Here is a diagram of the MSM molecule, with a sulfur atom in the central spot.

You'll remember that I had speculated in my theory of everything, that sulfur somehow played an important role in my health problems. But even though sulfur occasionally came up in my discussions with doctors, friends, and in my own research, I had not yet figured out how and why it was such a key player in this mystery. Finding sulfur in a substance that brought me a significant amount of relief was a nice confirmation that, in spite of the huge number of mistakes I had already made, I was indeed making a little progress with recovering my lost health and vitality. MSG was definitely not right for me, but MSM seemed to bring a significant amount of relief, and for both of these tiny breakthroughs, I was exceedingly grateful. And so, for the time being, I was content to take my daily dose of 10 grams of MSM per day.

Sometime later, I began taking MSM in powder form. It was easier for me to take one heaping tablespoon of powdered MSM than to swallow twenty pills. Plus, MSM in that form was far less expensive. But there was a downside. Because MSM is slightly alkaline, it has a bitter taste. That's actually being too kind, really. To be completely frank, MSM tastes terrible. But I found that if I chased it with some juice, I could get it down. It's been many years since this MSM discovery, and I still take this supplement occasionally for maintenance reasons. Living without debilitating back pain has taught me the value of taking my supplements faithfully—at least the ones that really work.

CHAPTER 7

# Not Eating "Just Anything" Anymore

My paradigm shift to a personal research-driven enterprise had yielded some very useful first fruits. I now had MSG in custody as a prime suspect with my food problems. This greatly encouraged me. Also, food labels no longer looked like hieroglyphics. I actually read and was starting to understand the chemicals listed on those labels. This knowledge helped me make the significant changes in my diet that I should have done years earlier. I humbly admit that I'd simply lacked the willpower to make those dietary changes before. But now, with a greater understanding of what MSG was and what it did to me, I found the will and the realization that this kind of food was just not worth it anymore. It was a hard but very valuable lesson to learn. I suppose that only people who have gone through food allergies can really appreciate how difficult it is to restrict what you put in your mouth.

Giving up my favorite store-brand cookies and chips and reading food labels was just the beginning. There was that huge elephant in the room known as restaurant food that had to be dealt with. There are no food labels on a restaurant menu. This is a problem for anyone with food allergies. Asking the waiter to make sure the steak is cooked on a clean grill doesn't work either. *Why do so many different restaurants make me sick? What do they put into their foods that makes my*

> There are no food labels on a restaurant menu.

*skin crawl?* I had no answers for these questions except MSG and "natural flavors," so for the moment, I was learning the art of discipline when it came to food.

I had a new and fresh resolve to stay true to my dietary restrictions. It was exceedingly difficult, but I worked hard not to succumb to cookout invitations at friend's homes. I was quite satisfied with these new self-imposed parameters on my eating habits. However, to the astonishment of no one but me, friends and family members did not share my enthusiasm for "just saying no" to food, particularly when it came to their food. This was another tough problem to deal with. Food allergies bring with them a type of social isolation. This took me totally by surprise.

Until now, I had not considered just how many social events are tied to food. It was just such a natural thing that I never even thought about it. All of this was changing. Now, when I was invited to join friends or family for a meal, I had to make some choices. At a restaurant, I could make the best possible menu choices and perhaps pay dearly for it later (which I had already resolved not to do); I could tag along for the ride and bring my own food (which is socially awkward); or I could simply decline the invitation (which is self-isolation). My chemical sensitivity had placed me in a lose-lose-lose situation in terms of eating out.

Having a meal at a family member's or friend's home was even more difficult. How do you gracefully say no to what is put on your plate? But I just had to stick with my new self-imposed eating restrictions. If I compromised, I would lose my resolve and end up right back where I started. After years of struggling with food, I desperately needed to stay on track with my commitment if I was going to win this battle. I was straddling a very fragile fence, and I knew it.

There is something both lonely and loathsome about chemical sensitivities and food allergies. When you finally come to grips with the notion that you can't eat just anything anymore, your life changes. This actually was a major life shift for me, more than I would have ever imagined. Eating food is so much more than simply getting necessary daily sustenance. Food is extremely social. It was only when I stopped eating any and every type of food that I saw the full reality of this social side of food.

I don't want to criticize my family or friends, because they were usually very sympathetic to my situation. But in all honesty, they simply didn't get it. Slowly, over time, I noticed that I was beginning to miss out on many social functions that I had normally been a part of—picnics, parties, weddings, a meal at a friend's house, or going out to eat at a restaurant. The social benefits of all of these gatherings were either gone or dramatically reduced. I never knew how much food allergies can make you feel isolated—even lonely at times—because they highlight a fundamental difference between yourself and other people. You know it. They know it. It's not a good feeling.

"Hey...let's all go out and get a pizza" doesn't sound so great anymore, because you are not sure you can eat that brand of pizza. You don't feel like lugging all your own food out to the restaurant because it makes you look neurotic. I found myself politely refusing those invitations more and more. And it only takes a few refusals like this before people stop asking you to come along altogether. Before long, you start hearing about how all of your friends went out to eat the other night, without you.

The point I am trying to make in all of this is that food is a huge part of society and social functioning. I never realized this until I could no longer participate in it. But my resolve with food was firm. I couldn't stop now. With regards to my friends and family members, I did not know if we could ever be back to the old way again. But I couldn't go back. I had to press forward.

Ironically, even though I was making some progress in my situation, I felt increasingly isolated by my circumstances. I realized I was a very different person than I had been only a few short years before, and I wasn't really sure if I even liked this new person.

CHAPTER 8

# By Any Other Name

I continued to dig into the research. I kept my focus on MSG, and it didn't take me too long to figure out that MSG and "natural flavors"—the two principal actors in my terrible drama—were not only very unhealthy to consume, they were often one and the same thing.

I wish I could accurately express my amazement and disgust as I researched the history of MSG. What MSG is, what it does, and why it is in so many foods—including (gasp!) certain brands of baby food is an incredible story. But I leave it to you, the reader, to do this research. For my part, I was faithfully reading labels now with a new understanding, and I found that the MSG alias of "natural flavors" is in a gigantic variety of foods. It seemed as if "natural flavors" was on almost every food label I read. But there is more. It turns out "natural flavors" is just one of the many aliases of MSG. As I really dove into the research, I counted nearly twenty different MSG aliases that are put into foods. Many of these aliases have rather impressive chemical names like hydrolyzed protein, autolyzed yeast extract, and soy protein isolate. If you are curious and would like to see more, do a simple web search on "MSG aliases" and examine the long and loathsome list for yourself. *So this was at least one reason why I was swelling up with foods that didn't list MSG or natural flavors on the label. I had been eating an MSG alias!*

> It turns out "natural flavors" is just one of the many aliases of MSG.

In spite of the rapidly growing list of foods that I knew I could not eat due to this MSG alias discovery, I remained positive. Things were making more sense. I had found another logical piece to the puzzle. A painful truth is always better than a smooth and convenient lie. At least now I had the truth. This allowed me to get more traction with some of my theories. I now had a much more comprehensive list of chemicals to avoid. The next step was another visit to my own pantry. It was time to take out the trash.

I rounded up all of the foods in my pantry that contained any of the various aliases of MSG and threw them out. Also, I wrote all of these aliases down on a list and kept them with me whenever I went shopping. After a short while, I began to see significant improvement concerning my allergic reactions to food. There were still times when I got caught in the MSG trap, but this was usually due to my own careless fault. One of the more hilarious episodes happened while I was in school.

I was taking graduate classes in Virginia at the time. During this particular summer term, I lived in a dorm room. I was disciplined with my diet, and if I did eat processed foods, I had my list of MSG aliases handy for quick reference. Since time is at a premium in graduate school, I spent most of my time either in class or studying. Eating was something that just needed to be done as quickly as possible. I ate the same cold cereal for lunch and dinner for a day or two, and then it happened. One morning I awoke with a monstrously swollen lip and cheek. I looked dreadful. I couldn't believe it was happening to me—not now! *How can I go to class like this? It looks as if I was just in a big fight...and lost. What caused this? I've only been eating cold cereal!* This particular brand of cold cereal has been around for about a hundred years. That is not an exaggeration. The cereal had only seven or eight ingredients, plus the added vitamins, and none of them were on my MSG alias list. Where had I gone wrong?

Well, I didn't have time that morning to figure it out. I needed to quickly think up a plan to fix myself so that I could get to class. Improvising on the fly, I found some rather large bandages and taped these over my grossly swollen face. I went to class, sat in the back, and tried to hide from the professor. But you can't hide your face in a classroom of twenty people.

I just looked weird and had to be content with that. Of course, people were very polite, and no one asked me any questions. My face was so swollen it even hurt to laugh. But I looked so ridiculous that I had to laugh in spite of the pain of it all.

After a day of classes, I got back to the dorm and went over all of the foods that I had eaten the day before. Everything checked out fine. I actually hadn't eaten much except that classic American cereal that consisted of milled corn, sugar, salt, high fructose corn syrup, malt flavoring, and just a few other ingredients. The cereal also contained a preservative common in many foods—BHT or butylhydroxytoluene. But I knew BHT wasn't the problem, because this preservative was found in many foods I ate, and it never caused swelling in me. This is not to say that BHT is entirely safe to consume, but I knew it wasn't the culprit. The only thing on this very short list of ingredients that looked weird to me was the malt flavoring. I had no idea what malt flavoring was, so I did some research on it. Well, you probably have already guessed it. Malt flavoring oftentimes carries or can be converted into MSG. Malt flavoring is an MSG derivative. One of my favorite cereals contained monosodium glutamate! I felt betrayed again. *Who can you trust for good food these days?* The answer is sadly obvious. You cannot trust food manufacturers, so you'd better get some knowledge concerning food additives, because you are on your own. The strange thing is that this breakfast cereal has been around for a hundred years, and it's highly doubtful anyone put MSG in their foods back then. The only thing I could think of was that the company must have changed the ingredients in this classic cold cereal sometime in the recent past.

I was on my own in Virginia that summer, but in a larger sense, I was on my own in terms of controlling and monitoring what foods I put in my mouth. Whatever trust I had in the food industry to provide me with good and healthy food was nearly gone. Blind optimism had dissolved into a cold cynicism. Food manufacturers and restaurant owners were not looking out for my health or my best interests. They were out for themselves. If that meant putting MSG or MSG derivatives into their products to sell more food to an unsuspecting and gullible public, they would. This was a sad revelation, and an admittedly pessimistic viewpoint, but I just could not escape the facts before me. And it wasn't just about food either.

During this time, I became very intent (some would say obsessive) on reading every sort of label imaginable. But this was for a reason. I sometimes found MSG or an MSG derivative in the strangest of places. Once I got burned with MSG in toothpaste. I'm not joking. Some brands of toothpaste carry an MSG alias. One evening I used a new brand of toothpaste without reading the label. I awoke the next morning with a fat lip. I went through the entire list of foods I'd eaten the day before and nothing was unusual. Finally I remembered that I had switched toothpaste brands. I checked the label of the new brand. It had carrageenan in it, which is a MSG derivative. *Have these people no shame? They put MSG in toothpaste?* It was almost too incredible to believe.

Another time we held a party at our home, and I woke up the next morning, swollen again. The same drill followed, going over everything I had eaten the day before. Do you know what the culprit was? *Ice cream.* The ice cream that we served at the party contained an MSG alias. I could go on with more tales of swollen woe, but you get the picture.

So which food manufacturers can you really trust to give you food that is really *food*, and not some chemically-laden concoction? That's a good question for which I have no answer. The best advice I have to this problem is for you to start educating yourself on the contents of food labels. I know of no other way out of this crazy maze.

CHAPTER 9

# Taking Stock and Getting Stretched

I was now four years into my mystery illness dilemma, and I had been making some progress in my understanding of my condition. In spite of these advances, I had no doubt that my overall health was continuing on a subtle, but decidedly downward slope. This was disconcerting, but at least I understood my situation better than I had before. The small victories I had experienced so far were encouraging, and even though my health continued to degrade, I felt that the rate at which this was occurring had slowed a little. I was carefully monitoring what I ate, and I was continually gaining information and an understanding of which foods caused issues for me and which ones didn't. I also had swelling episodes far less often, which was fantastic. But despite this apparent progress, it seemed as if I was getting progressively weaker. I think the best way to describe it is that I was aging at a greatly accelerated rate. I felt tired and frail much of the time, and I wondered if this was how it was going to be for me from here on out. If I put the various aspects of my health and overall functionality on a ledger sheet of assets and liabilities, I would have had far more entries on the liabilities side than on the assets side.

In terms of assets, I had discovered that I was allergic to monosodium glutamate. I had learned that MSG had a great number of aliases that were also to be avoided. I found great benefits in taking methylsulfonylmethane (MSM), a natural anti-inflammatory for my aching lower back. I was extremely determined to find the answers to my problems, and I was very open to trying new ideas and procedures. I also had money to test my theories, and I had very good insurance. Finally, my best assets were that I had my education and my faith. I knew that God had created the world of science, and He had the answers hidden in the world somewhere. I just needed to find those answers and then figure out how to correctly apply them. So I had many reasons to be optimistic, despite my admittedly miserable physical condition.

My liabilities at this juncture were fairly daunting. Although the discovery of the MSG issue had a definite positive effect on my allergic outbreaks, it was not a complete remedy. Even when I carefully avoided all of the MSG and MSG alias foods, I still had occasional outbreaks of swelling and rashes. I had no idea why this was happening.

And why had I suddenly developed food allergies about the same time that my back went out? Were the two things connected? It seemed as if they should be connected, but how?

And there were other liabilities. Sometimes my toes would feel numb. Sometimes the tops of my feet hurt. And of course, my lower back was stiff and aching much of the time, and it seemed as if I were always just one step away from throwing it out yet again. My lower legs were often restless, and at other times they felt very heavy. Furthermore, by anyone's estimation, I had a horrible immune system. I got sick with the flu every year, sometimes for several weeks at a time. Add to all of these problems the continuing issue of my sinuses. They were frequently plugged up, which made it extremely difficult to breathe at night unless I slept on my left side or went to sleep breathing through my mouth. The sad conclusion was that I was a miserable mess. But in spite of all of this, I tried to use this misery as a motivator to keep me going. I needed solutions to these problems, not a sympathetic ear for them.

> I was a miserable mess. But in spite of all of this, I tried to use this misery as a motivator to keep me going.

## TAKING STOCK AND GETTING STRETCHED

Having experienced a little progress on the allergy front, I started giving more attention to my back. This became my biggest and most immediate concern. It seemed like my lower back was getting progressively worse, no matter how much treatment it received. It was particularly sensitive to pressure, and sitting for long periods of time was just agony. I was still under chiropractic care and had gone faithfully for a few years now. At this point, though, I had been going only on an as-needed basis when my back went out.

Exasperated after many mornings of waking up with a back that seemed to almost be ablaze, I went to a pain management specialist. After his examination, the doctor concluded that my fifth lower lumbar disc (L-5) was inflamed and possibly bulging. He recommended getting an MRI (Magnetic Resonance Imaging) for confirmation. I was given the option for pain medication. I declined the medication, but I did agree to do the several different back stretches that the doctor demonstrated. I was told to apply ice to my lower back after doing the stretches. Well, the exercises and ice did help, at least for a little while. However, I suspected that I was still just chasing symptoms. *Why was my back so bad?*

I decided to get a second opinion, so I went to a homeopathic doctor who specialized in back issues. After an examination, this doctor agreed that I may have a disc problem. He also stated that I had another obvious problem that might explain why my lower back was constantly sore. He claimed that one leg was longer than the other. I'm not joking. This was one of the strangest diagnoses I have ever heard. It was another time when I felt that surreal feeling of entering a whole new dimension of weird. Thankfully I snapped out of my surreal stupor in time to listen to the doctor's directions. I was advised to wear a 4 mm heel lift in one shoe, at all times. If I wore several different types of shoes, he recommended putting one heel lift in each type of shoe. Very skeptical of this diagnosis and treatment but equally desperate to get some pain relief, I took his advice, especially since a heel lift cost only five dollars. After seeing perhaps a dozen doctors and paying tens of thousands of dollars—much of it out of pocket—finally I had an inexpensive medical bill.

For several months, I faithfully wore the heel lift and I did experience a certain level of relief. But as I continued under this specialist's care, I knew that my situation was not really improving. This doctor also utilized some chiropractic techniques and even acupuncture, but again, it seemed that this was just chasing symptoms. The nagging ache, discomfort, stiffness, and tenderness in my lower back continued. Eventually I went for the MRI, and sure enough, it proved conclusively that my L-5 disc was bulging. Grateful that it was only bulging and not herniated, I went back to the homeopathic doctor for treatment options. The doctor recommended what is commonly known as decompression therapy. I had no idea what this was, so he explained it to me.

At its essence, decompression therapy is basically taking a body and stretching it, particularly around the spinal area where the disc damage is. The idea was that by stretching the damaged L-5 area, the discs that are compressed can separate ever so slightly, thereby allowing the natural healing fluids of the body to enter the area and repair the damage. This doctor actually had a decompression machine in his office and had seen tremendous results from patients who had experienced issues like mine. This was good news. The doctor seemed very confident this procedure would work, and so, for the next twenty-seven days (excluding weekends), I had decompression treatments for approximately one hour each day. The first thirty minutes, I was placed on "the rack" as I called it, and stretched by tension wires. The rack was connected to a computer that tracked my time, progress, and the tension that was applied to my torso. The second thirty minutes, I was placed on ice and given electrical stimulation (using a device called a transcutaneous electrical nerve stimulator, or TENS unit) to accelerate healing.

After the twenty-seven days of decompression treatment, the doctor suggested that I gradually go back into my routine of heel lifts, stretching, and ice—all of which I faithfully did. After about four months, I can honestly say that my back seemed almost back to its old, *younger* self. By six months, it felt absolutely great. After a year, I was playing basketball again with little or no pain. This was incredible! After seeing so many doctors and getting little or no help, this homeopathic doctor was the first one who actually helped me recover some of my lost health.

Greatly encouraged by this success, I began seeing this same doctor in the hopes that he could help me with the food and chemical sensitivity issues I was also dealing with. Unfortunately, after many visits and many more dollars spent, this doctor was not able to help me with this. So it was back to the research and experimenting on my own. But I did this now with a lower back that was vastly improved. No longer in chronic pain, I felt as if a small portion of my life had been returned to me.

CHAPTER 10

# Clues from a Close Shave

Around this time of intensive rehabilitation on my lower back, I had an incident of sorts with my mouth. I started feeling swelling and pain in my cheek, but it wasn't due to eating anything that contained MSG. This pain was different. It felt like a toothache or large cavity, and it caused my cheek to swell. I went to my old dentist, had x-rays done, and received some bad news. One of my old root canals needed replacing.

Ever since I was a young boy, I disliked going to the dentist. All my life it seemed that, no matter how often or how hard I brushed, every time I went to the dentist, I'd have another cavity or two. I thought bad teeth just ran in the family because my mother had horrible teeth and a mouth full of metal fillings. I also had bad teeth. I had six metal fillings and four root canals, and now one of those root canals had gone bad. To make matters worse, my dentist told me he didn't deal with root-canal issues of this sort; I would have to see an oral surgeon. Since I was already in quite a bit of pain, I saw the surgeon within a few days. After a fairly quick examination, the surgeon confirmed my own dentist's diagnosis, and I had surgery almost immediately. Since I was only under local anesthetic, the surgeon talked me through the entire procedure as he was doing it. Were it not for the fact that it was me under the knife, I think I would have found this experience quite fascinating. I was extremely impressed with the surgeon's demeanor and professionalism, and I appreciated his calm and reassuring presence throughout the procedure. His main concern was to pull out the old root-canal apparatus without it breaking off inside my tooth's root. I was praying hard he would be successful.

Before too long, he announced he had found the source of my problems. He showed me a small post that looked like a tiny transistor, with two metal prongs sticking out of its bottom. He took his white glove and wiped those prongs with his fingers and said, "Do you see this gunk? This is actually corroded metal that was leaching into your body. If we hadn't taken this old root-canal post out of your mouth, it could have killed you!" With clamps and a suction still sitting in my mouth, I slurred this question:

"If this could have killed me, why did they put it in my mouth in the first place?"

"Well, back when you had this root canal put in, this was the popular material used at the time. Now we use much more advanced materials that don't corrode and leach into your system."

Well, I would like to say that this was a comforting answer, but it was not. Why in the world was material put into anyone's body that would later corrode like a rusty nail? And, according to the surgeon's own words, this stuff was deadly. I wasn't blaming this surgeon. In fact, I look back at this highly skilled professional as someone who actually saved my life. But I was extremely concerned as to why dentists would ever use materials that, under the guise of curing, could actually kill their patients. I was not afraid to die, but I have to admit I would have been ashamed to die if it was my own tooth that did me in.

> But I was extremely concerned as to why dentists would ever use materials that, under the guise of curing, could actually kill their patients.

This incident really bothered me. It also caused me to step back and really think about what was happening. Clearly, this latest swelling issue was due to the rusting prongs of an old root-canal apparatus, put into my mouth ten years earlier. Since I had been dealing with facial swelling for some time now, I realized that, while this was different from my allergic reaction swelling, there were some interesting similarities. I wondered if there was a connection between the rest of the dental work in my mouth and my chemical sensitivities. It seemed like a stretch, but there were similarities. In the meantime, I still looked ridiculously swollen, and I had to tell some people that this time the swelling wasn't due to something I had eaten—I had a bad tooth!

I also wondered if there could be a connection between the man-made materials in my mouth and my lower-back troubles. But after thinking about this for only a little while, this connection just seemed too far-fetched. But I wanted to keep an open mind about a potential connection between my bad teeth and my chemical sensitivities, so I looked into the matter further.

Over the next several months, things would open up in ways I never expected. Were it not for the fact that the information I obtained was backed by a huge amount of peer-reviewed scholarly research, I don't think I ever would have believed it.

CHAPTER 11

# Too Much Trust

I began focusing my attention on dentistry and dental practices. I had three old root canals in my mouth, a brand new one, and six metal fillings. I had a brush with death from an old root-canal post, according to the oral surgeon who extracted it, and I didn't want to go through that experience ever again. So, I began to research what these man-made materials in my mouth were made of, because I had far more questions than answers at this point. *What did I really know about metal fillings and root canal materials?* Almost nothing really, which now seems really strange. I had been having foreign substances placed in my body for decades, and I didn't even know what they were made of. Everyone in my family had metal fillings, and it was extremely common to see metal fillings in the mouths of most of my acquaintances. But I knew nothing about what the fillings actually were. Well, this was all about to change.

What I found in the research over the next few weeks shocked me and shook my confidence in the dental profession to its very foundation. I found books, scholarly papers, and even government studies that explicitly stated that metal fillings, the man-made material in my mouth, contained one of the most toxic elements in existence—mercury. I was speechless.

What I learned was that the silvery metal in my mouth, euphemistically called "silver amalgam," was actually over 50 percent mercury metal. Mercury! I'd had no idea that each of my six fillings contained this highly toxic metal. *Mercury had been in my mouth for decades! I had been swallowing mercury metal atoms ever since I was a boy!* I knew I had been swallowing the mercury because from time to time over the last twenty years, I had to have my fillings replaced. The old ones had "worn down." This was a revelation that was almost too incredible to even process correctly.

How and why would the medical and dental communities allow such a despicably foolhardy practice to occur in the modern age? Even the ancient Romans knew better than to mess with mercury. During the days of the republic and empire, the Romans actually used prisoners to work their mercury mines. That was 2,000 years ago. But in modern times, we willingly allow mercury to be placed in our mouths? This was outrageous.

I found study after study documenting the dangers of mercury amalgam fillings. Of course, I also found studies, many of which were sponsored by dental organizations, that stated that mercury amalgam fillings were inert—harmless. So which side of the debate was I going to believe? As a science teacher in public schools, I was fairly familiar with the major hazardous substances. Without a doubt, mercury was at the top of the list. There was no such thing as inert mercury. It was to be avoided at all costs. Ironically, about this time, our school district was actually doing an "all call" to every science teacher in the district to collect and properly dispose of all mercury thermometers. We were instructed to replace these with alcohol thermometers because the mercury ones posed a significant environmental and health hazard that the district wanted to avoid. Evidently, a neighboring school system was doing the same thing, but had not been as fortunate. I did not hear all of the details, but apparently a student accidentally broke a mercury thermometer in a science lab, and a small amount of mercury metal from the thermometer spilled to the ground. District administrators immediately closed the entire high school for two days so that this hazardous material could be cleaned up properly.

> This poison had been put into my mouth by individuals I trusted.

But what about me—*and countless others around the world?* I'd had this hazardous substance in my mouth since I was eight years old. Mercury was inside me! I was shocked, devastated, bewildered, and angry. I had no idea what to do at this point. No wonder I had thought my body was telling me it was being poisoned—it was! This poison had been put in my mouth by individuals I trusted. Was mercury behind all of my mystifying health problems? I had no idea, but I was going to find out.

In the months that followed, I devoured any reading material I could get my hands on concerning the dangers of mercury amalgam fillings. This material was not difficult to find. The internet is abounding with peer-reviewed scientific papers, books, websites, anecdotal stories, and government studies—both national and international—on the hazards of mercury toxicity. As I read just about every perspective there is on the subject, I found an entire spectrum of viewpoints. On one side are the dental and medical communities, who admit that people who have amalgam fillings will swallow mercury on a daily basis. However, they claim that these mercury amounts are very small and nearly harmless, and this mercury will pass through the body in just a very short period of time. On the opposite side of the spectrum are the conspiracy people, who claim that mercury amalgam is intentionally placed into the bodies of hundreds of millions of people as part of a diabolical plot to reduce world population and make an entire generation sick with diseases and conditions including cancer, autism, depression, and multiple sclerosis.

Since so many books and articles on the history and dangers of mercury amalgam exist, I will leave any further investigation of this to you. But I must warn you, the health profession's dangerous disregard over the hazards of one of the most toxic substances ever known will shake your foundations. It certainly did mine.

After my initial shock wore off, I had to determine my next move. I wasn't about to take any further chances with this so-called nearly harmless mercury amalgam. I knew enough about mercury from my chemistry background. The best way to deal with what I considered the most toxic substance on the periodic table was to leave it alone. Don't even mess with mercury. And yet, here I was with six mercury fillings in my mouth, most of which were at least ten years old! *Unbelievable.* I wanted these things out of me—now.

In terms of going forward, I had questions that required answering:

1. Did mercury have anything to do with my rapid fall from health over four years ago? If so, could this situation be reversed?
2. If mercury was at least partly to blame for my health demise, what was the mechanism by which mercury crashed my system?
3. How should I go about having my six fillings removed, and what should I do with my four root canals, three of which were quite old?

These were very important questions. I didn't have many answers at all at this point, but I knew I was onto something big. What exactly that big thing was, I wasn't sure. So I dove into researching mercury toxicity, mercury amalgams, and successful cases of amalgam removal. When I say I dove into the research, I am not exaggerating. I spent countless late-night hours on the web looking at blogs, websites, scholarly papers, journal articles, and government reports. It did not take long to realize that my worst fears were true. Mercury had been leaching into my system for over twenty years. Now it had all caught up with me. Virtually all of my symptoms—the food allergies, swellings, rashes, lower-back pain, general malaise and fatigue, sinus issues, frail immune system, and numbness in the extremities—all matched countless testimonies from other individuals with mercury toxicity.

During the first few weeks of this discovery, I was still somewhat skeptical of what I was actually reading. It was just too incredible to be true. But the more I read, the more commonalities I found. The same symptoms, the same stories appeared over and over again. Only the names of the individuals were different. *It couldn't all be a hoax, could it? Was I being duped yet again, or had this all actually taken place?* I came to the conclusion that there was just too much duplication in all of the data to dismiss it as a correlational coincidence. These were facts, and they couldn't be ignored.

Honestly, I was having a great deal of trouble processing all of this information and material, because I was really starting to be concerned with a new symptom that was rearing its ugly head: a rapidly failing memory. I had known for some time that my mental abilities were following a similar trajectory with that of my physical abilities. I knew that my ability to logically and correctly assess what was going on around me was slowly ebbing away. Unless I figured this whole thing out soon, I knew there would come a day when my mental abilities would erode to the point where it would be impossible for me to figure out this mystery. Worse, when I got to that point, I probably would be so apathetic about it all that I would not even care. This was now a race against time.

Thankfully, I was not at that point yet, but there were warning signs on the horizon. One such warning happened while I was teaching a high school chemistry class. Right in the middle of the class period, it suddenly dawned on me that I could not remember certain students' names. *That's weird. I've never had this problem before. What is going on with me?* I had to refer to the class roster just to make sure that I was calling on students by their correct names. This was totally out of character for me. Usually I had all my students' names memorized, even a hundred names or more, within a week or two from the start of the school year. But here I was now, months into the new school year, and I still could not remember certain students' names. This was bad, but it was not all.

I now found I had to do a significant amount of preparatory work before each class just to make sure I was familiar with the course material. And I had to consult my personal course notes frequently during the normal class time. This was also very unusual for me. Typically, I had the entire course material firmly memorized. But not anymore. It seemed now that some of the course material simply escaped me. I was having trouble processing even moderately difficult chemical calculations in class. Furthermore, I had to review the more complex calculations well in advance of the class so that I could demonstrate the calculations to my students.

I was losing my edge, intellectually speaking, and I knew it. But there was still more. I began to notice a growing gloom within me about the world in general. Little irritations became big irritations. Oftentimes, people in general just bothered me, and my usual optimism with people and circumstances was slipping away. I was edgy and restless much of the time. Sometimes I just wanted to escape the world's noise. I enjoyed being by myself far more often than usual, and I was becoming more interested in the virtual world of computer games, movies, and television than the real world. I didn't know it at the time, but I was slipping into the dark dimension of depression. But even through the deepening fog in which I lived, I knew the clock was ticking. Time was running out.

CHAPTER 12

# Frailty, Thy Name Is Mercury

I read every bit of information I could get my hands on concerning mercury toxicity. After this flurry of research, I no longer had a shred of skepticism that mercury was to blame for some of my health problems. Mercury was definitely a contributing factor, but was it the principal factor? Mercury is too powerful a chemical to not play a major role in destroying a person's health. I read numerous stories of mercury toxic people, and the parallels and similarities to my own situation were just too obvious to ignore. *I was mercury toxic.*

Despite my increasingly frail mental faculties, these months of research were extremely productive. I was finally getting some real data and real answers that made sense. This greatly encouraged me, and it gave me a much-needed boost to keep moving forward. As I conducted my research on the various effects of mercury poisoning, I was very surprised at how much of the data exposing the dangers of mercury toxicity is already out there, free for all to view and study. Many of these studies and analyses were highly critical of the three primary purveyors of mercury: the power companies that generate electricity in coal-fired plants (mercury vapor from burning coal), the dental community (mercury amalgam fillings), and the medical community (thimerosal in vaccines).

One piece of research I found said it all. *Mercury Exposure: The World's Toxic Time Bomb.* Produced for the United Nations, this essay discusses the damage that the worldwide use of mercury has done to entire populations. An even more detailed and accusatory report on the effects of mercury on physical and cognitive development was presented before the US Congress in 1997. *Mercury Study Report to Congress* is an exhaustive, 349-page peer-reviewed study that presents experimental data demonstrating the absolutely devastating damage that mercury can inflict on people.

> One piece of research I found said it all. *Mercury Exposure: The World's Toxic Time Bomb.*

These two studies were not written by fringe conspiracy theorists making outlandish claims. These studies came from the United Nations and the US government. I found these studies and others like them to be both compelling and convincing, and they had a powerful effect on my thinking about mercury. I also found some unexpected aspects concerning mercury that actually fit into the so-called theory of everything that I had created a few years prior.

I found that there is a strong connection between mercury metal and the element sulfur. In its natural form, mercury is found as an ore called cinnabar. The mineral cinnabar has the chemical formula HgS. If you are a little rusty with your chemistry, HgS is a molecule that has one atom of mercury (Hg) connected to one atom of sulfur (S). Cinnabar has a variety of uses, but all involve handling the highly toxic element mercury. History tells us that the ancient Romans used to have their slaves and prisoners work in the cinnabar mines because they knew cinnabar was dangerous. While this historical aspect of mercury ore was interesting, I continued to research its effects on a biological level.

The mere existence of cinnabar in nature proves that mercury has a strong attraction to sulfur atoms. Because of this attraction, when a living creature ingests mercury, this toxic element will leave the bloodstream and enter into tissues in order to bond with sulfur wherever it is found in the body. Sulfur is a main constituent of protein, so if you have mercury in your system, you will eventually find mercury in your protein. Mercury is such a strong element that it will often attempt to either take sulfur's place or bond to it in such a way that the biological benefits of the sulfur are nullified. Since sulfur is found in every protein and tissue type in the body, one would expect to find mercury in every type of tissue as well.

As ghastly as this sounds, I was actually very happy to discover just how pervasive mercury's influence can be in the human body due to its affinity for sulfur. Years earlier, I had suspected sulfur was a key factor in my mystery illness, and now I was starting to see how and why it was.

During my investigation, I found another powerful resource called *The Scientific Case against Amalgam*. This research piece, written by a dentist, exposes in stark detail the deadly effects of mercury fillings. It was written by someone who used to place mercury into his patients' mouths. Now this dentist is extremely active in trying to awaken a sleepy public to the dangers of mercury toxicity.

Included in *The Scientific Case against Amalgam* is an incredible study that came out of Canada several decades ago. Conducted during the 1980s, this Canadian study was simple in its construct. A single animal (a sheep) was given twelve mercury amalgam fillings that were tagged with a radioactive tracer. After this, the sheep was allowed to live for twenty-nine days, and then it was euthanized. An autopsy was conducted, and each key organ was analyzed for the radioactive tracer. The data chart here is the result of this study. As you can see, mercury was found throughout the sheep's body.

Mercury metal had literally filled the body of this poor sheep in only twenty-nine days! There was no doubt in my mind that the sheep was saturated with mercury in such a short time because of mercury's affinity for sulfur. It is highly irregular for poisons to be found in the brain, but the mercury was there as well. This was a significant finding because it shows that mercury can cross the powerful brain/blood barrier. Not many toxic substances have the power to do this. I was not ready to say that this explained why mercury-toxic individuals frequently show signs of mental dullness and depression in the early stages of the exposure, and outright insanity in the latter stages, but things were looking awfully suspicious.

I also found it interesting that there was a very low level of mercury in the sheep's blood, especially since mercury testing via bloodwork is a fairly common diagnostic practice. Apparently there is little in the blood that mercury has a strong affinity for, *so it leaves the bloodstream and opportunistically deposits itself in tissues throughout the entire body!*

This study also included some very interesting anecdotal evidence concerning the effects of mercury amalgam on overall health and wellness. Over 1,500 people answered a questionnaire that explored whether the removal of mercury amalgam fillings had improved their quality of life as they perceived it. While this is anecdotal evidence, it does not mean it is insignificant—particularly when many of the symptoms of these 1,500 people coincided with my own symptoms.

As I studied the data, I looked at my own known symptoms and charted them against that of the 1,500 people in the study. I found my symptoms repeatedly in the details. In fact, I saw so many similarities in this study to my own problems, I knew what my next move had to be. I had to get my mercury amalgam fillings removed—immediately.

Mercury toxicity was central to my health problems. I could not deny the evidence or retain any reasonable skepticism any longer. The United Nations report was true. Mercury is a time bomb. I had no doubt the people described in this report were just like me. They were going about their normal lives until a certain fateful day arrives, and the time bomb detonates. Suddenly, their health mysteriously collapses, and they have no idea why. This is what happened to me nearly five years ago. I was pulling that cart in my backyard when the time bomb went off, and my life has never been the same.

| Body Tissue | Mercury Levels (ng/g) |
|---|---|
| Whole blood | 9.0 |
| Urine | 4.7 |
| Skeletal muscle (gluteus) | 10.1 |
| Fat (mesentery) | 0.9 |
| Cortical maxillary bone | 3.6 |
| Tooth alveolar bone | 318.2 |
| Gum mucosa | 323.7 |
| Mouth papilla | 19.7 |
| Tongue | 13.0 |
| Parotid gland | 7.8 |
| Nasal bone | 10.7 |
| Stomach | 929.0 |
| Small intestine | 28.0 |
| Large intestine | 63.1 |
| Colon | 43.1 |
| Bile | 19.3 |
| Feces | 4489.3 |
| Heart muscle (ventricle) | 13.1 |
| Lung | 30.8 |
| Tracheal lining | 121.8 |
| Kidney | 7438.0 |
| Liver | 772.1 |
| Spleen | 48.3 |
| Frontal cortex | 18.9 |
| Occipital cortex | 3.5 |
| Thalamus | 14.9 |
| Cerebrospinal fluid | 2.3 |
| Pituitary gland | 44.4 |
| Thyroid | 44.2 |
| Adrenal gland | 37.8 |
| Pancreas | 45.7 |
| Ovary | 26.7 |

| Symptom Reported | Relief? | Me |
|---|---|---|
| Blood pressure issues | 54% | No |
| Urinary tract problems | 76% | Yes |
| Multiple sclerosis | 76% | No |
| Muscle tremor | 83% | No |
| Gum problems | 94% | Yes |
| Metallic taste | 95% | Yes |
| Sore throat | 86% | Yes |
| Oral ulcers | 86% | No |
| Skin disturbances | 81% | Yes |
| GI problems | 83% | Yes |
| Allergy problems | 89% | Yes |
| Bloating | 88% | Yes |
| Numbness | 82% | Yes |
| Chest pains | 87% | Yes |
| Irregular heartbeat | 87% | ? |
| Vision problems | 63% | Yes |
| Insomnia | 78% | No |
| Migraine | 87% | No |
| Irritability | 89% | Yes |
| Anxiety | 93% | Yes |
| Depression | 91% | Yes |
| Dizziness | 88% | Yes |
| Lack of energy | 97% | Yes |
| Lack of concentration | 80% | Yes |
| Memory loss | 73% | Yes |
| Thyroid problems | 79% | ? |

CHAPTER 13

# Skeptical Yet?

Some readers may take issue with the claims concerning the hazards of mercury that were brought out in the previous chapter. This is good, because frankly, these claims are in many ways incredibly indicting. You should be skeptical. *I know I was.* As I have said before, I encourage you to conduct your own research on the findings mentioned here.

While I found the data from the United Nations and the US Congress reports very useful, it was actually the data from the sheep study that truly opened my eyes to the dangers of mercury. Once I saw those tissue saturation numbers, I have not viewed mercury toxicity in the same way again. The sheep study was a simple, but powerful experiment that changed everything for me. Can one experiment be considered scientific proof of something? Scientific proof is found in repeating an experiment, not a memoir. I am telling my story, and I leave the rest to you. I am only sharing information, not giving medical advice. But if I did give some advice, it would be this: make sure you have hard data to drive your decisions. This is what I tried to do, because science can and should be reduced to hard data.

The studies presented to the US Congress, the United Nations, and the *Scientific Case against Amalgam* provided me with hard data that I could both understand and apply. I firmly believed that if I applied this and other information like it, correctly and without bias, I would regain my health. Well, eventually I did regain my health, but it was not without some resistance and objections from professionals in the health community. Because some of these objections and arguments are fairly common, I would like to address a few of them now.

First, people have argued that if mercury is as toxic as many say it is, why do dentists put this metal in people's mouths to begin with? This is an excellent question, for which I do not have an answer. When people ask me this, I suggest they look into the matter for themselves. I didn't waste time and energy trying to figure out why it happened or who to blame for it. I wanted answers. *How can this be fixed?* This was the question I was most interested in.

A second common objection that I have heard is this: Yes, mercury is toxic, but the form of mercury is actually the key. What dentists put into the mouths of their patients is *elemental* mercury. Because it is in its elemental form, it is mostly inert, and this inert substance passes harmlessly through the intestinal tract and out the feces.

This is an interesting viewpoint, because it is partially true. But it is not the whole story. Yes, the mercury put into people's mouths is elemental mercury, which is somewhat inert. If the mercury remained in this partially inert state, much of it should pass through the body relatively quickly. But remember the story of the high school that was shut down for two days because of a broken mercury thermometer? And what about that poor sheep in the *Scientific Case against Amalgam*? It took only a month for mercury to leach out of the sheep's amalgam fillings and literally fill its body with toxic mercury.

If elemental mercury passes harmlessly through one's system, why did the Romans use prisoners in their cinnabar mines instead of Roman citizens looking for employment? From all I read in the history books, being sent to the cinnabar mines was the equivalent of a death sentence. Cinnabar ore is a combination of a mercury atom and a sulfur atom. When this ore is heated, the mercury quickly evaporates and is easily inhaled.

The way I see it, arguing that the differing forms of mercury somehow protect people from the dangers of amalgam is just ridiculous, and anyone who uses this argument is either willfully ignorant of the chemistry or deliberately deceptive. Mercury is mercury. It is toxic in whatever form it is found. The only difference is in degrees of toxicity. There is no such thing as safe mercury.

The human body takes in the mercury and transforms its elemental form into an organic form of mercury by a complex chemical process. It may surprise you to learn that some of this destructive work is actually done by bacteria inside the human body. People are full of bacteria, and while most bacteria provide healthful benefits to the body, including aiding in digestion and the synthesis of vitamins, bacteria can also turn elemental mercury into its most dangerous form, methylmercury. This process is called "methylation," and it involves taking a mercury atom and attaching a single carbon and three hydrogen atoms to it. While all forms of mercury are to be avoided, this form is the most dangerous of all. Since people have loads of bacteria in their mouths, some of this bacteria will methylate the mercury atoms leaching from their fillings. This methylated mercury then mixes with a person's saliva and is swallowed. Even if some elemental mercury makes it all the way to the intestines, it can still be methylated by the bacteria living there. While the sheep experiment did show that a significant amount of mercury was excreted in the feces, there was far more mercury retained in the tissues of vital organs. This is the power of methylated mercury.

Another objection that I have often encountered is that pollutants are everywhere. People protest, "I can't change my life because of a little mercury in my mouth—or in my tuna. It's really not that big of a deal as long as it is in small amounts!"

I have to confess to you that this argument was pretty persuasive with me, at least at the beginning. Let's face it—we are constantly hearing about how bad certain foods are for us and how we need to avoid them. We've been warned of the dangers of toxins in our environment for so long, we are kind of numb to it all. Besides, it's only a small amount of poison that we are talking about, and changing one's diet because of a small amount of toxin is a major inconvenience.

This is a surprisingly shallow but fairly accurate excuse that people frequently give. We love food, particularly our comfort foods, and most of us will fight pretty hard in order to keep them. Of course, when we are backed into a corner and see our health falling apart, we finally surrender. Then we begin to make those serious dietary changes. I can only speak for myself, but I was more than just a little hesitant to change anything in my diet. However, once I decided that the pain of the status quo was greater than the pain of change, I started making the necessary changes. I was in such bad shape, I really didn't have much of a choice.

But even if you are not like me, and you hold onto your comfort foods with a much lighter grip than I did, you must remember that mercury isn't like any other environmental toxin. It is a uniquely powerful monster. It can invade every vital organ of your body, including your brain. I have seen more than just a few times that a major symptom of mercury toxicity was depression. If this was true, and I knew from personal experience that it was, then a person who is mercury toxic needs to get the problem corrected while they still care about it. Otherwise, there will come a day when the depression and apathy are so great, the person who is mercury toxic will not have the willpower to clean out the mercury, nor will they even care.

CHAPTER 14

# Plotting a Course

I compiled an extremely lengthy and disturbing list of many of the health problems that research had linked, either directly or indirectly, to mercury toxicity. It was a shockingly long list. I then categorized the list, which is shown below.

I knew mercury to be one of the most toxic elements in the world, but I had no idea how profound and far-reaching its health-destroying capabilities were. I also found in my research that mercury toxicity is uniquely tied to a person's particular genetic makeup. This was not surprising. Genetics play a powerful role in how people process, retain, and excrete many types of toxins. Mercury was no exception to this. Though mercury toxicity is clearly a global problem, genetics is the reason why not everyone on the planet has the same symptoms with their mercury toxicity. Because of genetic variation, mercury can cause a huge variety of health problems with virtual impunity. Working on a cellular level with only microgram amounts of mercury leaching from amalgam fillings on a daily basis, I imagine that finding the actual mechanism behind a person's chronic fatigue, or Epstein-Barr or multiple sclerosis—or whatever ailment a person is dealing with—would be exceedingly problematic.

The biochemical pathways mercury can use to cause any number of ailments is so complex and convoluted that it would be extremely difficult to trace a particular ailment back to a single point of origin. One day you find that you are diagnosed with multiple sclerosis, and you immediately link this supposedly incurable disease to mercury toxicity? Few would ever think this! If you find out you have MS or some other wretched superpower disease, the last place you would look for the cause of this disease would be in your own mouth.

## Mercury Toxicity

**Neurological & Cardiovascular**
Depression, detached from reality, brain fog, memory lapses, tremors, epilepsy, numb extremities, cramps, twitches, jitteriness, restless leg syndrome, fragile nerves, loss of sensory sensitivity, unexplained chest pain, unexplained tachycardia.

**Collagen**
Arthritis, frequent or constant pain, discomfort in joints; upper and/or lower back pain.

**Immunological**
Weakened immune system, ears, nose, and throat issues; autoimmune disorders, including MS, ALS, and lupus; Diabetes, eczema, psoriasis, certain types of arthritis, Epstein-Barr, cancer, AIDS.

**Hg Intake per Source:**

**Dental amalgam filling** (Hg vapor): according to the American Dental Association: 1.0–2.0 mcg/day
**Dental amalgam filling** (Hg vapor): according to the World Health Organization: 3.0–17.5 mcg/day (average 10 mcg/day, extreme 100 mcg/day)
**Fish** 2.4 mcg/day
**Non-fish food:** 0.3 mcg/day
**Air, water, food**: 3.09 mcg/day

**Miscellaneous**
Chronic fatigue, frequent urination, bloated feeling after eating, recurring constipation, ringing in the ears, metallic taste in mouth, TMJ, headaches after eating, hormonal irregularities, low sex drive, suicidal thoughts, airborne allergies, food allergies, severe digestive problems including Candida, Crohn's, and other digestive flora-related illnesses. Mercury toxic individuals may excrete mercury via sweat, saliva, feces, urine, and semen. Mercury can move freely through fetal blood supplies and breast milk, causing potential danger to unborn and nursing children.

I began to look at mercury as if it were a professional thief. Mercury sneaks in imperceptibly, steals and destroys at will, and then hides in undetected places. It does this with extraordinary efficiency, erasing all evidence of its presence, and escapes without detection.

Besides raw genetics, the other factors involved in mercury toxicity were much more straightforward, such as mercury dosage amounts and time of exposure. If the numbers from the World Health Organization were correct, I had accumulated a significant amount of mercury during my lifetime due to my amalgam fillings. This was a rather depressing revelation. But, trying to remain optimistic, I was glad to at least be on the right track with my investigation.

So what was my next step? I had six mercury amalgam fillings in my mouth. Each filling added to my daily accumulation of poison. This had to stop. But once this was done, how would I get my tissues cleared of all the deeply embedded mercury? I imagined myself similar to that poor sheep, except that I'd had mercury fillings in my mouth for nearly twenty-nine years, not twenty-nine days! And remember, after only twenty-nine days, the sheep had mercury in its brain, lungs, stomach, thyroid, kidneys, intestines, and so on. Just the thought of this made me angry, disgusted, and somewhat helpless. I felt trapped and victimized by mercury. It was like a bad horror movie where I was the monster that arises from the laboratory table and asks its maker, "What have you done to me?"

I knew I had a very long road ahead. There would be no quick fix. Instead of being frustrated at the magnitude of the big picture, I tried to focus on taking just the few small steps that I knew I had to take.

In looking back over everything I had already tried, it was now clear why all my attempts to get better were abysmal failures. Although the treatments and protocols I undertook provided some symptomatic relief, true causal relief had always eluded me. Now I knew I had been doing very little, if anything, to get the toxic mercury out of my body. In fact, I was actually accumulating more mercury each day as it leached from my fillings. Maybe all of those years of swallowing mercury had brought my internal systems to a final tipping point, until it all crashed down upon me that day in my backyard, pulling the garbage cart. This seemed like a reasonable theory, but I had no way of knowing for sure. The one thing I did know was that I had no time to waste.

The first step was to stop the daily influx of mercury metal. I started researching the extraction of amalgam fillings, and I found that dentists who specialize in this sort of thing are known as biological dentists. I am a total outsider in terms of the professional dental community, but from all that I learned concerning biological dentistry, the men and women who practice mercury-free dentistry are considered sort of as rogue professionals by the mainstream dental community. *Rogue professionals. Ah, these were just the type of people I was looking for.*

I decided to have a biological dentist do the extractions because as far as I could tell, biological dentists took the most conservative precautions available to ensure that their patients were not given more mercury (swallowing tiny pieces of metal or inhaling mercury vapor during the drilling) throughout the extraction process. I read the American Dental Association's advised practices for amalgam removal, and I found the reading quite revealing. One thing that stuck out in my mind was what dentists actually do with the old mercury fillings that they extract. The American Dental Association (ADA) has stated that old mercury fillings are considered hazardous waste and need to be placed into special receptacles upon removal. Yes, you read that correctly. According to the ADA, the amalgam filling is "safe" until it is removed from your mouth. Then it is considered hazardous waste and an environmental threat that must be stored in a specialized container. So in other words, what is in the mouths of hundreds of millions of people around the world is not even suitable for the regular garbage can. *Unbelievable.*

Anyway, I found a biological dentist in my area, and I made an appointment for the initial consultation concerning the extraction of all six amalgam fillings and for their replacement with nonmetal materials.

The next step would be figuring a way to measure my progress. From all of my research, I found that the human body works constantly to rid itself of toxins. I wanted to find a way to quantitatively measure my improvement after my fillings were removed. It wasn't just enough to ask myself, "*Well Chris, how are you feeling today? Do you feel better today than a week ago? In what way(s) do you feel better?*" That is considered qualitative research, and although I believe there is significant value in qualitative research, I wanted hard data, based on numbers. I needed something I could chart, graph, or plot quantitatively that would parallel the improvements I was hoping to feel qualitatively.

In order to do this, I had to choose one of three options for measuring mercury content in the body: blood analysis, urinalysis, or hair analysis. I decided against blood and urine testing for several reasons. First, from all I could ascertain, neither blood nor urine accurately measures the long-term body burden of mercury. As was found in the sheep experiment, mercury seeps into tissues rather quickly, so I wondered what significant amounts of mercury found in either blood or urine would really be telling me. Was the mercury going into the tissues, was it coming out of the tissues, or was it simply going around and around? Second, it seemed that I needed something that showed long-term trends—and that is what a hair analysis provides. This was not going to be a quick fix over a six-month period. Mercury imbeds itself in tissues, and it has a strong affinity for sulfur. That means the mercury will make its way into proteins, which are found everywhere in the body, just as the sheep experiment demonstrated. Furthermore, not only did I prefer the way the hair analysis tracked long-term data, I also liked the fact that I could do this in my own home and interpret it for myself.

No more frequent doctor visits, no more misdiagnoses, and no more friendly "Well, you are not responding to that treatment as well as I would have liked, so let's try something new." I was done hearing all of that.

> I needed something I could chart, graph, or plot quantitatively that would parallel the improvements I was hoping to feel qualitatively.

If you are unfamiliar with toxicity testing through hair analysis, as I was, I suggest you consider the book *Hair Test Interpretation: Finding Hidden Toxicities*, by Dr. Andy Cutler. I love this book because of its depth, perspective, and amazingly wise and intuitive nature. Dr. Cutler is not a medical doctor. He is a chemist who was himself a victim of mercury poisoning. He has no apparent axe to grind against the medical or dental professions, but he, like me, was desperately seeking answers and not finding them in the standard medical community. Dr. Cutler is also a huge proponent of hair analysis as a diagnostic tool, and the substance of most of his work is based upon the hair analysis results of hundreds of people who have or had mercury toxicity.

Many doctors and organizations are against using hair analysis, citing its supposed unreliability for testing of heavy metals, but their objections seemed flimsy to me. I thought that either those who objected to its usefulness either didn't fully understand how to interpret a hair analysis report, or they had another agenda that was, frankly, not hidden very well.

For example, there are plenty of articles published on how hair analysis is not useful for measuring heavy metals, but these same people and organizations loudly praise the virtues of using a hair analysis test for controlled substances and drug abuse. In essence, they are stating that using hair analysis—which can be done in the convenience of one's own home to test for mercury, arsenic, or aluminum—is not accurate, but using a hair analysis that is completed in a doctor's office to test for cocaine, amphetamines, or cannabis is accurate. This just did not make any sense to me. A toxin is a toxin, and the body will use whatever avenues it has at its disposal to excrete the toxin. These avenues include feces, urine, sweat, breath, and hair. But just to be safe, I decided to test drive the hair analysis as a diagnostic tool. If I was wrong about the efficacy of the hair analysis test and got some crazy-looking random data after a few hair-sample reports, I would find a new diagnostic tool. If, however, the data seemed to follow a particular trend or correlation, I would stick with the test throughout the duration of my detoxing.

Things were moving along fairly rapidly now. I had my dental extraction consultation appointment date, and I had a quantitative diagnostic tool ready at hand. I had just one more major decision to make. What method would I use to induce my body to expel the mercury that was embedded throughout its tissues? This was a pretty big question to consider. The technique commonly used today is called *chelation*.

Basically, a chelating substance grabs onto a toxic metal—whether it be mercury, lead, nickel, aluminum or some other toxic chemical—and binds itself to it. By binding to the toxin, the chelating substance makes the toxin either inert or less reactive, then it uses the body's normal pathways to excrete both itself and the toxin. It didn't take long for me to find that the market is literally flooded with chelating substances and protocols that claim to assist in the detoxification of heavy metals.

After a significant amount of research, I decided on one particular chelating supplement that was specifically designed for the metals found in amalgam fillings. Furthermore, this chelating substance was designed to excrete the toxic metals through the intestines via the feces, not through the kidneys using urine. From all I had found, excretion through the feces is the best way to get rid of toxins because it follows the body's natural design. Most of the waste we excrete goes through the intestines, so it seemed logical to chelate heavy metal toxins using this excretion pathway.

I had already spent thousands of dollars on supplements and had gotten very little in return except large credit card bills at the end of the month. Now I was looking at spending more money again on supplements. But this time, things were different. Now I was going to be taking supplements specifically designed not to put nutrients into my system, but to pull dangerous chemicals out. This was a huge shift in my strategy. Once all of the bad chemicals were taken out, my system would then be able to actually benefit from the good supplemental nutrients I was putting in. This was something that I hadn't thought of before, but it really seemed to make sense now. Getting healthy requires first taking the bad things out of your body before putting the good things in. Yes, I would be taking some nutritional supplements as I was chelating. But I felt that I would only get the true benefit from these nutritional supplements—and from the normal food in my diet—when my system was first cleared of the toxins it had been accumulating for decades.

After five long years, I finally had some real direction and momentum to my cause. I had a good plan, and I was enthusiastically going forward with it. There was no turning back now.

CHAPTER 15

# Taking that First Step

All long journeys begin with a single step. Now it was my turn. I was ready to begin my personal detox protocol to rid my body tissues of the mercury metal I had been accumulating almost my entire life. Ironically, my plan for accomplishing this seemingly monumental task was actually quite simple:

1. Get baseline data.
2. Have mercury amalgam fillings removed.
3. Begin taking chelation supplements.
4. Experiment with other detox protocols as I became aware of them.
5. Periodically send in hair samples to measure progress.

I would use the information from my first hair analysis report as my baseline data. I was fairly confident this data would be an accurate reflection of my body chemistry and overall toxicity. Dr. Cutler's book, *Hair Test Interpretation: Finding Hidden Toxicities* was an excellent resource for reading the hair analysis. Given the clarity of the book's directions, I was reasonably certain I could correctly interpret the data from a hair analysis report. To be perfectly candid, although the biochemistry is very sophisticated, the hair analysis report itself is fairly easy to interpret.

After I had the baseline data, I then had to take at least one trip to the dentist to have the mercury fillings removed. It wouldn't make sense to start detoxing mercury if I was concurrently adding mercury to my body on a daily basis. Following the removal of the fillings, I would begin taking the chelation supplements, and journal my progress. Periodically, I would send more hair samples to the lab in order to determine my progress. *Would there be a significant numerical improvement in the hair test results over time, and would that improvement match how I was feeling qualitatively?* I hoped the answer to both of these questions was yes, but of course, nothing was certain at this point. I gave myself a little haircut and sent my first hair sample to the lab. The results came back in a few weeks, and this became my baseline data. Many hair analysis reports have two sections, one for the bad elements and one for the good elements. Here is the data from the bad side of this first hair report.

| **POTENTIALLY TOXIC ELEMENTS (My Baseline)** | | | | |
|---|---|---|---|---|
| | RESULT µg/g | RANGE | PERCENTILE 68th | 95th |
| Aluminum | 25.0 | < 12.0 | | |
| Antimony | 0.054 | < 0.080 | | |
| Arsenic | 0.11 | < 0.120 | | |
| Bismuth | 0.040 | < 2.0 | | |
| Cadmium | 0.029 | < 0.150 | | |
| Lead | 0.750 | < 2.0 | | |
| Mercury | 0.30 | < 1.10 | | |
| Uranium | 0.090 | < 0.060 | | |
| Nickel | 1.100 | < 0.40 | | |
| Silver | 0.22 | < 0.10 | | |
| Tin | 0.84 | < 0.30 | | |
| Titanium | 0.78 | < 1.00 | | |
| **Total Toxic Representation** | | | | |

The phrase "potentially toxic elements" refers to the harmful elements that were in my system at the time of the test. The numbers indicate the levels at which they were found in the hair sample. I firmly believed these were the main chemicals behind at least some of my health problems.

Black lines that reach into the 95th percentile column meant that I was in the extreme range of toxicity. The hair analysis report is actually a statistical and probability report of how your body chemistry compares to everyone else's. If you are in this 95th percentile range, you are in an exclusive class of toxicity, along with the other unfortunate 5 percent of the people who have an extremely high level of a particular toxin. This is bad—very bad. As you can see from this report, I had extremely high amounts of nickel and tin in my system. While this was disturbing, it was not unexpected. Mercury amalgam is just that—an amalgam. It is a combination of mercury, silver, tin, nickel, copper, and a few other elements. The four root canals that I had also contained toxic metals, including a significant amount of nickel. So even from a cursory overview, this first hair analysis report seemed to make a great deal of sense to me. The high toxic levels certainly were not what I wanted to see, but unfortunately, they were what I expected to see. On a positive note, the fact that I was high in the exact toxins that are found in mercury amalgam and in root canal material spoke to the usefulness, even accuracy, of hair analysis as a credible diagnostic tool.

Having said all of this, the data showed that I definitely had work ahead of me. Those long black lines had to get shorter. I didn't want even one element to be in the middle 68th to 95th percentile range, and I had five, with one element—nickel—past the 95th percentile. My goal was to be in the lowest range with all of these elements, and if it was possible, to not even have a line on the chart at all.

If you look at the bottom of my baseline data, you will see a summative line entitled "Total Toxic Representation." I estimate I came in around the 75th percentile in terms of a total toxic representation. From just a sheer statistical and probability point of view, I was sicker than approximately

74 percent of the other people who have taken a hair analysis, or at least this is how I looked at it. Many people don't like hair analysis specifically because it deals with statistics and probability. But for my part, the hair analysis suited my purposes just perfectly. I wanted baseline data, and now I had it. I had a summative measurement in the total toxic representation number, and I had real quantitative data concerning various dangerous elements that were currently in my body. And, most conveniently, I had done this all from the comfort of my own home.

As a chemistry teacher, I was simply fascinated with the elements that were found in my own hair. The elements shown on the hair analysis report looked like a Who's Who list from Poison Control. *Aluminum*—a toxic metal linked with Alzheimer's disease. *Arsenic*—a toxic element sometimes used in rat poison. *Nickel*—a toxic metal linked to heart and kidney damage, as well as hormonal imbalances. There was the slow-killing *lead*—linked to many health problems, including Alzheimer's, dementia, and liver and kidney failure. And, of course, there was *mercury*, which has been linked to more diseases and debilitating conditions than I cared to even think about. On the hair analysis report, the mercury level looked relatively small compared to some of the other toxic levels. But I knew this was part of the deceptive nature of mercury. From what I understood in the research, mercury is not excreted in the hair in large amounts because it quickly and powerfully binds to other tissues in the body. To make matters worse, mercury strongly reduces the body's ability to excrete other toxic chemicals. So even though mercury looks like a pawn in this toxic chess match, it is actually the queen of toxicity in disguise.

> The elements shown on the hair analysis report looked like a Who's Who list from Poison Control.

I could go on about this first hair analysis report, but you can see for yourself that it is a rather bleak picture. This first report was bad, but I imagine it could have been far worse. In fact, I have seen far worse reports, and I'll show you one of these in a later chapter.

I was making good progress, and now I needed to find a way to get the hair analysis numbers smaller and the lines shorter, and to do it as quickly as possible. I had my baseline data with real numbers. This was my rock bottom, or so I thought, and now I just had to reduce those numbers and the lengths of those lines. After the removal of my mercury fillings, I would use chelation supplements, as well as any other detox protocol I could think of, to pull the toxic elements from my body. Then I would get another hair analysis to check on my progress. If I was successful, the lines should get shorter and the numbers should get smaller. This whole plan was actually quite straightforward. But would it work? To be perfectly candid, I had my doubts. But there was so much work to do right now, by sheer momentum I kept moving forward.

From looking at my baseline data, I knew what I needed to do next. I had to make a few easy but necessary lifestyle changes. If you look back to my baseline report, you will see that my aluminum levels were extremely high—somewhere near the 85th percentile. This was way too high. Dr. Cutler had mentioned that mercury disrupts normal mineral transport in the body. He called this disruption "deranged mineral transport." Obviously my aluminum excretion pathways were quite deranged. How did this happen?

Imagine for a moment all of the specific routes that vitamins and minerals take inside your body. Mercury has the unique ability to disrupt the traffic on these biological highways. But that's not all. Mercury also has the power to damage the highway itself. This is one reason the arsenic and uranium levels were so high in my baseline report. It wasn't because I had a habit of playing with rat poison or radioactive waste. These toxic elements were in my body because we all live in a toxic world. Poisons are all around us. The problem with me was that my body could not excrete these toxins as fast as I accumulated them from the environment. This was all due to deranged mineral transport, driven largely by mercury metal. I knew that

I could not control most of the toxins to which I was exposed, particularly those from the soil, water, or air. But there were toxins that I could control. One of these was aluminum.

The first thing to go was my aluminum cookware. It went right into the trash. As a teacher, I never did a chemistry experiment using an aluminum container—only glass. Heating aluminum would allow aluminum atoms to leach into the mixture and potentially spoil the experiment. I imagined cooking with aluminum metal was the same thing. Stainless steel was also suspect, because it contains a significant amount of nickel, which like aluminum, is also considered a toxic metal. I found reasonable evidence to suggest that nickel would leach into food that was cooked in stainless steel. So, that cookware also went into the trash. Even if the amounts of nickel and aluminum that leached into my food were considered trace amounts, I wasn't taking any chances. It was much better to err on the side of caution, particularly when my baseline amounts of aluminum and nickel were so ridiculously high.

After doing a little more research, I also discovered that aluminum is found in several different brands of antiperspirants. Some of these I used. *Okay...check that item off my grocery list from now on. No more aluminum-carrying antiperspirant.* If you think about it, it is actually shocking that aluminum is even in the stuff that we put on the open pores of our skin. No wonder aluminum gets into the blood supply so easily—the skin pore doors in the underarm areas are wide open!

Of course, the manufacturers of aluminum-containing products will say that their products are safe, that the levels of aluminum are so small they are harmless, or some other line intended to placate a worried customer. Companies that sell health-compromising products are masters at engineering the consent of the public. I was not taking any chances though, especially when the fix—changing cookware or changing antiperspirants—was so easy.

I wanted to conduct sound science experiments on myself using standard methodologies. I wanted to keep as many variables the same as I could, but I also wanted to get better...*immediately*. So, despite all my efforts to utilize sound methodologies, I broke the rules on numerous occasions. I made several variable changes concurrently over the course of the next several years.

If I wanted to conduct a perfect experiment, I would have eliminated aluminum intake and made no other significant lifestyle or experimental changes for three to six months. After this time, I would have sent out another hair sample to see what changes had occurred in my hair analysis aluminum levels. Then I would have repeated the procedure for another three to six months and compared the data again.

This is excellent science in a procedural sense, but I am a person, not an experimental variable. I wanted to get well, and not wait. So I included changes with multiple variables and then looked at the results and tried to work backwards to find the causal agents to credit—or blame. I didn't have the luxury of a ten or fifteen-year window of time for experimentation utilizing double-blind procedures. So even though my application of the scientific method during my detoxing was admittedly sloppy at times, I did it because I knew time was at a premium.

CHAPTER 16

# Skin for Skin

After receiving my baseline hair sample data, I was ready to have my mercury fillings extracted. Following my initial consultation with Dr. Michael, my biological dentist, I knew I had made the right decision in choosing both biological dentistry and this doctor. Dr. Michael was just the sort of person I wanted and needed. He was extremely thorough, experienced, and cheerful. I really appreciated that in particular, because I have always dreaded going to the dentist. Dr. Michael assured me that every precaution would be taken to ensure my safety throughout the mercury extraction process. These safety precautions are extremely important—so much so that I believe Dr. Michael and the oral surgeon who earlier extracted my corroded root-canal posts literally saved my life.

I was a newcomer to biological dentistry, but I was very impressed with what I heard and saw in this dental clinic. Apparently other people in the area felt the same way. Because of the extremely busy schedule of Dr. Michael, my dental extraction date was nearly four months away. Though Dr. Michael advised me that six amalgam fillings may be too much mercury removal for a single sitting, I insisted on doing them all at once. I wanted this whole thing over in one sitting, and the quicker it was done, the better. Looking back, this was probably another mistake of mine. Any mercury extraction process will necessarily bring about some level of mercury ingestion, no matter how many precautions are taken. I had read numerous reports from professionals highly experienced in mercury extraction, and the research was fairly unanimous that the process is hazardous. Taking a toxic element out of the tooth cavity is dangerous to everyone present in the room. The dentist's spinning drill bit immediately vaporizes the amalgam metal, and breathing in mercury vapors is not something anyone should do. Furthermore, the mercury amalgam may crack or chip as it is being drilled, and the patient may swallow tiny fragments of it. The whole procedure was a risk. But I knew the risk was worth it. I really had no choice in the matter. Not doing anything to remedy what I was certain was at the core of my problems was not a solution—it was capitulation.

> Not doing anything to remedy what I was certain was at the core of my problems was not a solution—it was capitulation.

My extraction date was still a few months away, but I was eager to get started with my detox immediately. So I decided on a detox protocol that seemed far more ostentatious than it actually was. Years earlier, a homeopathic doctor that I greatly respected had begun using far infrared technology in his clinic as a detoxification tool. This far infrared technology was applied in the form of a sauna.

I know what you are thinking. *Are you serious? A sauna...for detoxing?* That's what I thought too, but after looking into it, sweating out toxins looked to be an effective—not to mention relaxing—way to eliminate poisons. I knew that the major excretion pathways of feces and urine would be the main modes of eliminating the internal toxins, but I was intrigued with the technology surrounding this seemingly extravagant way to detox through the skin. Sweating out toxins has been used as a detox protocol for millennia. The far infrared (FIR) sauna was just the twenty-first century's version of this ancient detoxification modality. And when I considered the fact that this was a detox protocol that could be done without taking any more pills, I was sold. So, for a cool $3,000, I bought and installed a portable FIR sauna in my garage.

By now you might be wondering if this decision contradicted what I had spoken of previously. Yes, I knew that the human body has two principal paths of waste excretion—the intestines and kidneys—and I needed to clear and strengthen those pathways, not circumvent them. But skin was a third pathway, and what if I could combine detox protocols that addressed each of the three main excretion pathways simultaneously? Would not this be an extremely powerful and rapid mode of detoxing a poisoned body like mine?

I did not have a good detox for the intestines or kidneys yet, but I was convinced that the FIR sauna would do nicely for the skin portion of the equation. Make no mistake, this was not an impulse purchase. I did my due diligence before pressing the check-out button on the FIR sauna website. From all I could gather, far-infrared radiation penetrates the skin and breaks up the fat cells just under the skin's surface. I had known for some time that the body stores toxins in fat, and this seemed like a convenient, comfortable, and relaxing way of detoxing the largest organ in the body—the skin. Oh, did I mention that *fun* was also a driving factor? I was able to do a detox protocol that I actually enjoyed! True, the sauna was not cheap, but after spending thousands of dollars on treatments and supplements that had done very little good, sweating profusely in a sauna was one detox protocol I knew would work.

CHAPTER 17

# Under Mike's Drill

Several days before the extraction date, I met with Dr. Michael once more for x-rays and a final consultation. During this time, he talked me through all of the steps that he would take to ensure I was protected as much as possible from the mercury and other toxic metals that would be released during the extraction process. I felt that I was putting my life in his hands, and after speaking with him several times before the big day, I wanted as much assurance as possible that I would make it through the procedure intact. I also watched and listened to Dr. Michael very carefully. He was definitely the sort of doctor I needed: highly skilled, knowledgeable, and fast. When the extraction day finally came, I was both excited and nervous to get this whole thing over with.

When all the protective measures were in place—a highly ventilated room, powerful suction for picking up both amalgam fumes and tiny amalgam pieces, a rubber dam to collect the large pieces of metal, an oxygen gas mask, protective eyewear, and several pills of activated charcoal already in my stomach—Dr. Michael began the extraction procedure. To be completely honest, with all of these protective measures in place, I was not nervous at all. The procedure lasted several hours, but it was ultimately uneventful. New ceramic fillings were put into place, and before I knew it, I was at the front desk setting up an appointment for a follow-up consultation and inspection.

The whole process was actually far easier than I had envisioned, but I imagine that was due in large part to the tremendous skill and experience of the doctor. A short time later, I had an excellent post-extraction consultation and a pre-op consultation for my next dental extraction.

Yes, there was still more work to be done. You see, after a significant amount of research and after personally consulting with a detoxification expert in the dental field, I had decided that even though what I had done to eliminate mercury from my teeth was a good thing, it was not enough. I still had four root canals, and three of them probably had metal posts because they were so old. I wasn't sure about the types of metal involved, but it was a good bet that nickel was part of it. The nickel metal had to go. After coming so far, I did not want to repeat history.

What good would it be to have the mercury extraction procedure if I willingly left some other toxic metal like nickel in my mouth? Metals corrode. They also ionize, and ions generate free radicals. Free radicals destroy health. So I wanted the metal out. I needed it out—all of it. This was particularly important considering my previous history and the narrow escape described earlier.

Dr. Michael agreed to perform the procedure, which he later did with outstanding precision and professionalism. And then it was over. Finally, after considerable expense, time, and energy, I was completely metal free.

Of course, this was not true on the cellular level, and that was where my real work was about to begin. But finally, after more than twenty years, I was no longer soaking in regular amounts of toxic atoms that leached from my fillings or from aging root-canal posts. Yes, I had mercury from my vaccinations, and mercury from environmental and food sources as well, but just being able to stop the huge daily influx of metals leaching from fillings in my mouth felt very, very good.

CHAPTER 18

# The Look

Things were moving along nicely. The man-made materials were finally removed from my mouth. I had hair sample baseline data, there was a wonderful FIR sauna operating in my garage on a regular basis, and I was taking chelators to remove the metals that were embedded in my tissues. I was off to a very strong start. I was also convinced my plan to get the bad chemicals out of my body before trying to put the good chemicals in was an absolute winner. Thus, besides taking the chelators and a very good multivitamin, there was not much else I was taking in terms of supplements. Furthermore, I was becoming increasingly comfortable with doing my own research, and as I continued to do so with some experimentation, my knowledge and experience with detoxification grew. This growth affected my confidence, and I was starting to see and feel that my original goal might indeed be possible—*I could regain all those lost years due to bad health.* However, all of this progress had come at a price, and it only partially had to do with money.

I had clearly broken away from the traditional health-care establishment, and was openly critical of it in certain areas. This raised some eyebrows with friends and family members. I'd had my silver amalgam fillings removed. This raised more eyebrows, especially with people who still had mercury fillings in their mouths. I was doing detox strategies on my own without being under the constant supervision of a medical doctor. Still more eyebrows went up. Conducting my own detoxification strategies without traditional medical supervision seemed very arrogant and audacious to some, and utter foolishness to others. I regularly faced questions, skepticism, disapproval, and *the look*. Do you know what I mean when I say "the look"? It's that face that people give you when you are doing something they disapprove of, but they don't want to appear as if they disapprove of it.

"So, Chris," a friend says, "I understand you've had some very strange health issues over the last several years. I am very sorry. What is the name of your doctor? I know of someone who could give you excellent care."

"Thank you. Actually, I have already seen far too many doctors. I've been doing a significant amount of research on my condition, and I'm experimenting with a few different detoxification protocols on my own." Then I brace for impact. Here comes the look.

After I received my doctorate—in education, not medicine—I got the look less often. Instead, I heard a new line, typically spoken behind my back, just slightly above the threshold of hearing.

"There goes Dr. Mercury. He's always talking about how dangerous those silvery fillings are in your mouth. But you know, his doctorate is not in medicine—it's only in education."

*Sigh*. I was not an expert in detoxification medicine, nor had I pretended to be one. But after five long years and well over $50,000 in out-of-pocket expenses, I felt that the so-called experts weren't experts at all—at least not in the areas in which I needed them to be. Facing the subtle criticism of the look and the gossip was nothing compared to what I had already gone through.

I felt that I was waging war against my own body. Now that I finally had some direction and purpose, I wasn't going to let the criticism of others stop or even slow me down. Besides, I wasn't planning to punish my body with any bizarre detoxification protocols (although I did come close at times) that had no basis in research. True, I was fully prepared to use my renegade physical form as a laboratory of sorts. I was doing *experiments*. That sounds a bit sinister, but the only malevolence I really wanted to display was against the toxins. The toxins had to go, and by getting rid of man-made materials in my body, I had taken an excellent first step.

> I felt that I was waging a war against my own body.

From all that I understood in the research, if the protocols I was doing were actually working, the first thing that would happen would be mobilization of the toxins. When toxins are liberated from tissues, they have an initial negative influence on the person doing the detoxing. These liberated toxins affect the good mineral transport and absorption pathways. This is a fancy way of saying "side effects." I knew I might feel worse before I would feel better, and similarly, the data might look worse before it looked better. But the toxins had to be mobilized from their hiding places, which very likely were the fatty tissues all around the body.

Mobilization would come first, and then the binding, and then the excretion. That's where the chelators would come into play. Chelators are chemicals specifically designed to bind to toxins. Since I was no longer swallowing mercury atoms that leached off the amalgam fillings, I was hoping that my body's own natural detoxification mechanisms would sluggishly reawaken and work synergistically alongside the chelation supplements and my FIR sauna treatments, to effect real positive changes in my health. This was my strategy. But although I thought this strategy was a good one, I still had many questions.

What if the chelation supplements I was using, specifically designed for amalgam filling metals, did not effectively bind to the toxins? Or what if the binding did take place successfully, but my body could not effectively excrete the toxins quickly enough? What would my body do with the newly liberated mercury, aluminum, arsenic, or any other toxin that was flowing through my system instead of being excreted? From all I could find in the research, the newly liberated toxins would over time settle back (reabsorb) into the body's tissues. Then I'd be back to square one.

Reabsorption is a very common occurrence with detoxification. The body tries to excrete the toxins, but if it can't within a certain amount of time, it has to try to hide the toxins all over again. The body cannot tolerate toxins freely flowing through its system, bonding to proteins, disabling enzymes, killing cells, and releasing or stealing electrons from other systems—basically starting their own free radical free-for-all.

Reabsorption was a serious concern that I had no immediate answer for, but I was hopeful that the qualitative and quantitative data would be so encouraging going forward that this concern would be unnecessary. Even if the sauna and chelation supplements were completely useless, I still had one strong advantage in my favor. I was no longer daily adding to my mercury metal intake. According to the ADA and the World Health Organization, the amount of mercury that will leach off just one filling into the saliva is approximately 1 to 5 micrograms per day. If I did my chemistry calculations correctly, just one microgram (one millionth of a gram) contains approximately 300,000,000,000,000 atoms of mercury. Just one atom of mercury is all that is required to destroy or deactivate a living cell. *One atom.* That is the power of mercury. Before my dental extractions, I was adding millions of mercury atoms to my body with each and every swallow. No wonder I was so sick! But that was all behind me now, and even if every detox protocol I tried from this moment on was an absolute failure, I was certain I would see at least a small improvement in my health.

CHAPTER 19

# The Terrifying Theoretical Leap

About this time in my personal detox journey, I took a theoretical leap of sorts with an idea that I have never heard or read of before in any of the research. Perhaps the reason I had never heard of it before was because it was so off base that no one would even entertain such a notion. Or perhaps—and honestly, I wish I was wrong about this—the theory was just wild enough to be true. But the theoretical leap was just that—a theory, and it could be false. But if it was false, it sounded so very much like the truth. With all this being said as a way of introduction, please allow me now to share with you the origin of my terrifying theoretical leap.

I had been collecting information on mercury toxicity for over a year, and the pile of data was really starting to accumulate. The information came from a variety of sources, many of which were quite prestigious, including the US government's EPA and FDA, the World Health Organization, and the American Dental Association. One day, I was pouring over the material, looking for commonalties and trends. The technical term for what I was doing was called "triangulation." This involves gathering data from a variety of sources and looking for common threads that can be found running through each source. By triangulating data, you increase your own scope and understanding of the data while simultaneously increasing the probability that the data is both reliable and accurate. I tried to link my growing pool of data with the data from the sheep experiment, as was shown in chapter twelve. I later also read of another study using sheep. In this study, a female sheep was given mercury amalgam fillings with a radioactive tracer. The scientists then milked the lactating sheep and found radioactive mercury in the sheep's milk after only six hours from the implantation of the amalgam fillings! These studies, and others like them, demonstrated the awesome and invasive power of mercury. This invasive power was dramatically evident in the first sheep experiment. It took only twenty-nine days for mercury to leach from the sheep's fillings and find its way into virtually every vital organ of the sheep's body, including the brain. If you look again at the chart in that chapter, you will notice that nearly nineteen nanograms of mercury found its way into each gram of the sheep's frontal cortex. Nineteen nanograms per gram seemed like a very large concentration of mercury in the brain for only twenty-nine days' worth of exposure. This told me that mercury can circumvent the powerful brain-blood barrier, which is highly unusual, and it can bypass this barrier very quickly. *But if mercury can get around the brain-blood barrier, and find its way into a mother's milk supply, could mercury also circumvent the vitally important fetal-blood barrier?*

    I dove into the research on this very important question. Sure enough, I found study after study from US and world health agencies stating that mercury does indeed cross the fetal blood barrier. Even the American Dental Association admitted that this occurs, but of course, the ADA quickly added that the amounts that crossed over the barrier were not detrimental to the health of the child. I disagreed with this. It seemed impossible to me that the ADA could prove the mercury that crossed over was not detrimental to the developing child's health. One atom of mercury can potentially disable an entire cell. If only one atom of mercury can disrupt a cell, clearly no amount of mercury can be considered safe.

    If mercury can reach an unborn child, that was danger enough. And once a baby was born, there was still significant danger from the baby's own mother! It took only a few hours for mercury from the sheep's mouth to make it into the nursing milk. If this was true with sheep, it was doubtless true with humans as well. I saw no compelling reason why one mammal would have a more advanced defense system against heavy metals than another. But if this was true, then mothers who have amalgam fillings would be feeding their own babies milk that was tainted

## THE TERRIFYING THEORETICAL LEAP

with mercury! This was almost too incredible to believe. What a horrid logical leap this was.

But I remained skeptical. This couldn't be true. I kept digging in the research to find some way, some mechanism or biochemical pathway that would nullify this idea. I began with a simple web search with the terms "pregnancy danger with amalgam fillings" and read and researched until I nearly got sick with dread. Blogs, studies, scholarly papers, and testimonials all seemed to scream that this fear of passing mercury from mothers to their children was grounded in fact and reality. *Human mothers with mercury in their mouths give mercury to their unborn children via the fetal blood supply. This means that babies are born with mercury already embedded in their tissues, and these tissues would be in some of the most sensitive areas of the body, including the brain.* And it gets worse.

Because this is the fetal blood supply, mercury is introduced to the developing baby before most of its normal defenses against toxins even exist. The baby is exposed to mercury virtually at conception and is largely defenseless from this toxic onslaught. This is why an unborn baby is far more vulnerable to the deleterious effects of mercury than a grown adult. Furthermore, if a baby develops in a womb with mercury present, a vast array of devastating congenital conditions could potentially arise from this toxic exposure. Worse still, this exposure would probably never be traced back to its true point of origin because it happened so early in life—and because we have all been told that amalgam fillings are safe.

My head was swimming with this chilling scenario And the nightmare wasn't over. I wasn't done theorizing. There was still one more logical step to take.

*What if the mercury passed from mother to child is generational?* There was no compelling reason to dismiss this frightening theoretical leap. It seemed logical. Mothers who had mercury, passed at least some of this mercury into their unborn

> What if the mercury passed from mother to child is generational?

children. When these children are born and grown, the females passed the mercury—some of the very same mercury atoms that they received from their mothers—on to their own children!

In terms of my personal history, this all made sense; albeit in a grim sort of way. If the theory was correct, I was actually *born* with mercury poisoning. I got this mercury from my mother, because she had mercury fillings in her mouth at the time of my birth. As she carried me in her womb, I was given mercury-laced blood for nine months. After I was born, she nursed me with mercury-laced milk. I had no idea what my grandmother's teeth were like, but I knew her generation was also exposed to mercury in dentistry, because it has been used in the United States since at least the 1930s. I couldn't say for certain, but it was a good bet that my maternal grandmother also had mercury fillings. So theoretically, I could have had trillions and trillions of mercury atoms in my body that came from my maternal grandmother's body. This was possible because mercury circumvents the fetal blood barrier through the generations of the maternal bloodline.

This could be one reason why vaccinations with thimerosal (a mercury-based preservative) are so controversial. Perhaps the reason both sides of the debate are so vocal is because both sides are, at least in one sense, correct. The amount of mercury in vaccines is small, but it is not insignificant. It is about the same amount that would leach from a single mercury amalgam filling over a twenty-day period. But what if the children getting the vaccines already have mercury in their systems from fetal blood and breast milk? This new introduction of mercury metal might be all that was needed to push the child's mental and physical health over the proverbial cliff. Who is to say? The mercury vaccine debate has been going on for a very long time, but as far as I knew, the idea of generationally transmitted mercury has never been a part of this debate.

If mercury could be transmitted through the generations, a frightening reality on a macro level began to take shape in my mind. If this was possible—and I had not found any argument or evidence to contradict it—then a majority of the population in the United States, and a large percentage of the world's population would have health problems either

# THE TERRIFYING THEORETICAL LEAP

directly or indirectly related to mercury toxicity. It was as if mercury metal was now infused into the human gene pool. We were born this way. Do you now see why this is a terrifying theoretical leap? But there is still more.

In terms of the current dental practices in the United States, mercury amalgam fillings have fallen out of favor. Today, people typically prefer the white ceramic fillings to the silvery-colored mercury ones, but not because they are told mercury is a toxin that will leach into their bodies on a daily basis. Most people choose the white ceramic material simply because it is less noticeable and more aesthetically pleasing. But people who have never had a mercury filling in their life could still be full of toxic mercury. It depends upon the dental health of the mother, grandmother, great-grandmother, and perhaps even great-great grandmother! It is the maternal line that requires attention, not the paternal line, because the mercury is passed through fetal blood and breast milk. The point is that mercury was introduced into the human population generations ago, and its effects could be just as destructive, if not more so, as time progresses. It no longer matters whether you ever had mercury fillings or not.

At first glance, this seems counterintuitive. *How could mercury be more destructive as the generations pass and not less?* You would think that the mercury would just work its way out of the system as it passes through the generations. Wouldn't each subsequent generation be less and less affected by the mercury? This is an excellent question that I considered for some time. Eventually I concluded that subsequent generations of people would actually be more in danger of mercury toxicity than earlier generations, and I had three reasons for theorizing this.

First, I knew of the tremendously attractive power mercury has for sulfur. Mercury leaves the blood system very quickly and bonds to sulfur wherever it can find it. This was shown graphically in the sheep experiment. Clearly, mercury does not leave an adult person very easily. It clings to proteins in tissues with a very strong chemical attraction. If this was true with adults who have a fully functioning immune system, I suspected this would be even more pronounced in a developing child.

Secondly, mercury is present at conception. Long before the body has built a mercury defense system, mercury metal is present in the body, busily doing its destructive work. Mercury is a thief. Mercury in a developing child is similar to allowing the thief into a building before the alarm system is built. By the time the alarm is built and switched on, much of the damage has already been done. A child fed a fetal blood supply laced with mercury would have mercury in the deepest tissues and most fundamental areas of its body. The mercury would be systemic. Therefore, the second generation of mercury-toxic individuals would most likely have weaker and less efficient mercury-excretion mechanisms as they grow into adulthood than first-generation mercury-toxic individuals. The third generation would have an even weaker and less efficient excretion system than the second generation, and so on.

The third reason I had in mind was birth order. When a mother is carrying mercury in her mouth, she will necessarily give increasing amounts of mercury to successive children because the mother's own mercury accumulation is higher as she grows older. I was the fourth of four children. My mother had several mercury fillings at the time of my birth. Incidentally, I often heard my mother complain about her teeth as I was growing up. It was a constant problem throughout her adult life, and by the time of her death, I believe my mother had metal fillings on every tooth in her mouth with the exception of her front incisors. If my theory was correct, I received the most mercury of all my siblings, because I was the youngest. With this revelation of sorts, suddenly my severe health problems made much more sense. Although each of my siblings could have been displaying some symptoms of mercury toxicity, none of my family had the serious chemical sensitivity issues that I was dealing with.

In all of this theorizing, I have stated nothing concerning genetics. I did this for a reason. I knew genetics played a role in mercury absorption and excretion because I had seen it so often in the research. Some people have a genetic predisposition toward excreting toxins more efficiently than others. This is probably one reason why mercury toxicity can manifest itself with such a huge variety of debilitating conditions. But genetic influences on mercury absorption and excretion was far beyond my area of control. My main and immediate concern was that mercury was in the human bloodline—my bloodline. I was second-generation mercury toxic, possibly even third-generation mercury toxic. And if my theory was correct, how could I reverse its effects on me?

As was my pattern, I had to give my theory a name. I had no doubt that mercury toxicity was indeed generational, so I called my new theory "generational mercury transmission," or GMT. This theory had three simple tenets:

1. Mercury is transmitted via the fetal blood supply and breast milk.
2. Mercury is passed on to generations through the maternal bloodline.
3. Birth order plays a significant role in mercury toxicity, with younger siblings being at a potentially greater risk than older siblings because of the mother's higher mercury burden at the time of their birth.

Even though GMT was still just a theory, it was an extremely disturbing one. And unfortunately, it was a theory that I could not find any research or reasons to dismiss it. After thinking about it for some time, I actually was thankful that I wasn't sicker than I already was. Mercury is such a toxic element, and it had been inside me since the day I was conceived. What a mess I was in, and I still wasn't finished. The likelihood of GMT being true forced me to take one more logical step. This was where all of my theorizing and experimenting suddenly became extremely personal.

*What about my two children? Are they mercury toxic?* I had a daughter who was three years old at the time, and a son who was five. Neither had received much in terms of vaccinations when they were born because even before I knew of any of this, my wife and I were extremely cautious about giving our infant children any shots. We also did not feed our children fish—not because we were aware of the tuna-mercury connection at the time, but because we simply did not eat much fish at home. But my two children did have a mother who had six mercury fillings at the time of their births, and a maternal grandmother who'd had mercury fillings since she was a young girl. If all of my theorizing was even a little correct, both of my kids were third-generation mercury toxic. They seemed like healthy kids, but I had to be sure. I needed more data.

I decided to give them both a little haircut, then I sent their hair samples to the lab for some hard data. If the news from the lab was good or great, with no bars to the end of the chart, then my whole terrifying theoretical leap was probably far more science fiction than science fact. But if the news from the lab report was bad...well, I was just not sure what the next step would be. Hopefully the lab reports would be great, and then I would gladly dismiss my theory of generational mercury toxicity as just that—a theory with some potential merit, but without any concrete evidence to support it.

CHAPTER 20

# Light the Fuse

Up until this point, I was serious with my research, but it was just *my* research about me. I experimented with supplements and some interesting protocols, and I consulted with, and was evaluated by, more than a few health care professionals. And I made plenty of mistakes along the way. But I could afford to make those mistakes, because it was just me. When I received my kids' hair analysis reports back from the lab, this perspective totally changed. My terrifying theoretical leap was now not just some crazy theoretical notion—it had support. The data from the hair analysis reports from both of my kids looked absolutely terrible. In fact, their data was worse than mine. *I literally felt sick to my stomach.* Suddenly, detoxing took on a whole new level of urgency, because I knew my children were at risk. I still could not conclusively say that my theory of generational mercury transmission (GMT) was correct, but I could confidently state that this new data failed to disprove the theory. I had to assume that my theory was correct. This was the only responsible decision I could make. I simply had to find a solution to this toxicity problem and implement it while my kids were still young. If I waited until they got older, it might be too late.

My first step was to do some comparisons. When I considered my baseline data, I knew it didn't look great. With a total toxic representation around the 75th percentile, I suppose things could have been far worse. But when I compared my baseline data to my son's baseline data, things suddenly got much worse. My son's total toxic representation was approximately the same as mine—and he was only five years old! I was stunned. This was absolutely horrible news.

## POTENTIALLY TOXIC ELEMENTS (5-Year-Old ♂)

| | RESULT µg/g | RANGE | PERCENTILE 68th    95th |
|---|---|---|---|
| Aluminum | 29.0 | <12.0 | |
| Antimony | 0.041 | <0.080 | |
| Arsenic | 0.073 | <0.120 | |
| Bismuth | 0.28 | <2.0 | |
| Cadmium | 0.044 | <0.150 | |
| Lead | 0.26 | <2.0 | |
| Mercury | 0.05 | <1.10 | |
| Uranium | 0.040 | <0.060 | |
| Nickel | 0.71 | <0.40 | |
| Silver | 0.32 | <0.10 | |
| Tin | 0.15 | <0.30 | |
| Titanium | 2.1 | <1.00 | |
| **Total Toxic Representation** | | | |

Like any father put in this situation, I wanted my kid's toxicity numbers to be as low as possible. Long black lines on their toxicity report was something I certainly did not want to see. Frankly, I wanted my GMT theory to be completely wrong. But if it was correct, my two kids were at least third-generation mercury toxic, and possibly fourth. I could think of no other major sources of mercury transmission other than fetal blood and breast milk. Neither of my kids received much mercury in terms of vaccinations. The five-year-old had had only one vaccination, and the three-year-old had none at all. This ruled out thimerosal as a mercury source. Environmental mercury in the air and soil did not seem a likely source that could do this level of damage. I couldn't think of any food sources either. As I said before, we almost never ate fish of any kind. The only source of mercury that I could think of was generational, coming from my kids' mother and maternal grandmother.

Here is my three-year-old daughter's data. Her toxic element levels were outright insane. Her total toxic representation was literally off the chart. These levels were far worse than her brother's levels. But if my theory concerning birth order was correct, these higher levels were to be expected. My daughter's body was built with fetal blood and breast milk that was saturated with two more years of mercury than her brother, so finding baseline data that was this bad actually made sense.

| POTENTIALLY TOXIC ELEMENTS (3-Year-Old ♀) | | | | |
|---|---|---|---|---|
| | RESULT µg/g | RANGE | PERCENTILE | |
| | | | 68th | 95th |
| Aluminum | 38.0 | <12.0 | | |
| Antimony | 0.17 | <0.080 | | |
| Arsenic | 0.043 | <0.120 | | |
| Bismuth | 0.84 | <2.0 | | |
| Cadmium | 0.21 | <0.150 | | |
| Lead | 1.3 | <2.0 | | |
| Mercury | 0.14 | <1.10 | | |
| Uranium | 0.098 | <0.060 | | |
| Nickel | 1.100 | <0.40 | | |
| Silver | 17 | <0.10 | | |
| Tin | 0.61 | <0.30 | | |
| Titanium | 5.0 | <1.00 | | |
| Total Toxic Representation | | | | |

I was devastated. Parents want the very best for their kids, and this includes excellent health. I had been struggling to regain my own lost health for the past five years, and now I was slammed with a whole bunch of new data that screamed mercury toxicity in my own kids. If there was an upside to any of this, it was that I had this data early in the lives of my kids. This gave me time to get things under control before their health conditions worsened.

I didn't spend too much time on the specific, individual toxic levels. Again, this is where many people get confused and frustrated with the hair analysis report. They look at levels like these and wonder how and why silver or titanium are so ridiculously high. I didn't bother with this too much. The critical issue to keep in mind is that if a person has mercury, their internal mineral transport system will be deranged. This will result in the person having a very difficult time excreting certain toxic elements. The hair levels accurately reflect the body's metal burden. If the mineral transport network is functioning normally, these lines would be much shorter. But if the mineral transport pathways are deranged, due largely to mercury, the body simply cannot excrete the silver, titanium, nickel, or whatever toxic element you choose, like a normally functioning body could.

My goal at this point was not *why*, but *how*. How could I proceed in order to get these toxins out of my kids right now? If I was going to make a mistake in any of this, I wanted to err on the side of caution, so I needed a protocol to be both fast and safe. I got moving, all the while keeping in mind the golden rule of scientific experimentation: *safety first*.

To begin with, I assumed that the lab data was correct and accurate, both for my actual body burden of toxins and for that of my two children. If I was wrong and the data was not accurate and my kids were actually far healthier than their lab reports indicated, I reasoned it was still a win-win situation. My detoxing strategies were going to be so safe that the kids could only benefit from it anyway, even if they were

> Because my kids were little, I knew I had some time to fix this situation. But I also knew that I had no time to waste.

relatively toxin-free. If however, the data was accurate, the detox strategies would hopefully work quickly to reverse this serious problem. Because my kids were little, I knew I had some time to fix this situation. But I also knew that I had no time to waste.

CHAPTER 21

# Breaking Through

I was now about halfway into my twelve-year detoxification journey. At this juncture, my own protocols became somewhat secondary to those of my kids. This detour lasted nearly two years. I still pursued my own detox strategies, but I focused most of my energy on my kids. I saw their needs as far more pressing than my own. Even though I undoubtedly had a greater toxic burden because I was older, I also had far more weight and fat in which to carry those toxins. My kids had neither of these things going for them. They were still growing, and I wanted to get as much of the toxic junk out of their bodies as possible while they were still young.

> If I could safely detox them at a young age, I felt their body's own natural detoxification mechanisms would be revived, and would finish what I started.

If I could safely detox them at a young age, I felt their body's own natural detoxification mechanisms would be revived, and would finish what I started. The goal was to do this safely, effectively, and quickly. If it could be done in the proper manner, I believed their physical and cognitive maturation would not be seriously affected by insidious metals, like mercury, working inside them. But mercury wasn't just going to leave on its own. I had already learned that lesson the hard way.

So, over the next two years, I gave my kids the same mild over-the-counter detox chelating supplement that I was taking, but in dosages appropriate to their ages and weight. Thankfully, this particular chelating substance came in liquid form as well as in pill form. Having the chelating substance in liquid form made the entire process so much easier. My kids happily drank their "vitamins" every day. After about a year and a half of chelation, my kids seemed just as happy, and maybe even a little bit healthier, than they were before. They were both prone to seasonal colds, but after sixteen months of chelation, their immune systems seemed a bit stronger. This was my observation, and honestly, it could have simply been wishful thinking. I needed quantitative data to provide solid evidence that their "vitamin drink" was really working, so I sent in a hair sample from my daughter to the lab for analysis. I chose to test my daughter's hair first because of the wretched numbers in her baseline report. If the chelation protocol was actually working, I wanted to see it in her data first.

| POTENTIALLY TOXIC ELEMENTS (5 Year Old ♀) | | | |
|---|---|---|---|
| | RESULT µg/g | RANGE | PERCENTILE 68th    95th |
| Aluminum | 25 | <12.0 | |
| Antimony | 0.027 | <0.080 | |
| Arsenic | 0.049 | <0.120 | |
| Bismuth | 0.091 | <2.0 | |
| Cadmium | 0.061 | <0.150 | |
| Lead | 0.85 | <2.0 | |
| Mercury | 0.27 | <1.10 | |
| Uranium | 0.16 | <0.060 | |
| Nickel | 0.36 | <0.40 | |
| Silver | 0.14 | <0.10 | |
| Tin | 0.25 | <0.30 | |
| Titanium | 2.1 | <1.00 | |
| Total Toxic Representation | | | |

The results came back from the lab in a few weeks, and I breathed a huge sigh of relief. The test results showed *significant* reductions in toxin levels. This data was just what I needed to see. I was not even close to claiming victory in the war on toxicity, but a small battle had been won.

| Toxin | Original Level | After 16 Months | % Increase or Decrease |
|---|---|---|---|
| Aluminum | 38.0 | 25.0 | 34% Decrease |
| Antimony | 0.17 | 0.027 | 84% Decrease |
| Arsenic | 0.043 | 0.049 | 14% Increase |
| Bismuth | 0.84 | 0.091 | 89% Decrease |
| Cadmium | 0.21 | 0.061 | 71% Decrease |
| Lead | 1.30 | 0.85 | 35% Decrease |
| Mercury | 0.14 | 0.27 | 92% Increase |
| Uranium | 0.098 | 0.16 | 63% Increase |
| Nickel | 1.10 | 0.36 | 67% Decrease |
| Silver | 17.0 | 0.14 | 99% Decrease |
| Tin | 0.61 | 0.25 | 59% Decrease |
| Titanium | 5.0 | 2.10 | 58% Decrease |

Shown here are the numbers measured against those numbers from my daughter's baseline data, which had been collected approximately sixteen months earlier. Nearly all of her toxin levels had decreased, with the exception of mercury. But this was expected. From all that I understood about chelation, mercury levels typically rise before they fall. Mercury was being liberated from all of its little hiding places in my daughter's body. Now in a mobilized state, the mercury was released into the bloodstream and some of it makes its way into the hair, so the hair sample level of mercury necessarily rises. I fully expected mercury levels to fall in subsequent tests, and I also expected the levels of the other toxins to continue to fall as my daughter's internal mineral transport system grew stronger and less deranged.

So my daughter, now five, not only appeared healthier, but I had real numbers and real data to back up my observations. *What a relief.* Like any parent, I wanted to give my kids the absolute best chance for a great future, and vibrant health was a part of that. My son, now seven, had also experienced fantastic improvement. But I wanted to share with you my daughter's data because her baseline numbers showed a far greater initial toxicity, and now I had data showing the dramatic nature of her improvement.

This was a huge victory. Finally I was starting to see the great toxic iceberg begin to melt. I was excited to see where this was going, as the mild detoxification path that I had taken with my kids would continue into the years ahead. I did not deviate too much from this extremely simple protocol with the exception of three elements that I added later on to clean out their thyroid glands.

Throughout this process, I always kept to the philosophy that because my kids were still small, the supplements that they took had to always be at extremely conservative dosage levels. My kids were too small and precious to *experiment* on. But for me—well, that was another matter.

During the sixteen-month window that I was giving chelation supplements to my kids, I took almost the same supplements that they did, but in dosages appropriate to my age and weight. To my utter surprise, I did not get nearly the same results that my kids did. In fact, I wasn't sure I was getting any benefit from the supplements at all. I didn't feel any better, and my hair analysis reports during this same time window were also largely unchanged. This was strange. *How is this possible? The kids are obviously getting significant benefits from these supplements, while I am not. What is going wrong?*

After some research and reflection on this apparent inconsistency, I eventually came to the conclusion that I was just too toxic systemically to get the same benefits that my kids were getting. The only thing that I could think of was that my absorption levels of the chelation supplements must be woefully inefficient. Taking a mild chelator that contained chlorella, cilantro, alpha lipoic acid, NAC (N-Acetylcysteine), and a few other substances worked extremely well for my kids, but not for me. And simply increasing the dosage amounts of these supplements didn't work for me. Either I was too toxic for these conservative measures, or I just needed more time for them to work. *But that was just it—I didn't have more time. I needed something to work now.* Clearly, the only solution left for me was to find a far more powerful protocol than just taking a mild chelating substance and doing regular FIR sauna treatments. But what was it? I had tried so many supplements, ranging from easy-to-find foods, to exotic herbs, to ridiculously expensive pills and protocols. I saw very little qualitative or quantitative improvement from any of these things. So, I went back to researching and tried to figure out where I had gone wrong. There must have been something important that I had missed—something I was not doing. I had seen and experienced firsthand the futility of just taking supplements blindly and hoping for the best. Now I needed something bigger, and better.

After still more research, I decided to focus my attention on detoxing a specific organ. I had been working on the intestines with herbs and other supplements for some time now, and even though I didn't experience any problems with this like chronic diarrhea or constipation, I didn't see any real improvement with my symptoms. I still had my food allergies, chemical sensitivities, and all of my other problems. So I gave up on trying to fix my intestines and decided to move upstream. I turned my attention to the liver.

Focusing on the liver seemed logical, because the liver is the body's main detoxification organ. The liver is also a blood filter. I knew from my working on my old car that filters need frequent cleaning if they are going to do their job properly. Well, the liver is the human body's main filter, and so much more. The liver has a huge number of responsibilities, not the least of which is to construct chemicals needed to detoxify the body and to assist in digestion—two areas that I had definite problems with. I had also found that mercury attacks the liver and hampers its ability to conduct its detoxification duties.

Now think about that for a moment. *Mercury attacks and weakens the one organ whose job it is to remove mercury.* When I really grasped the significance of this fact, a light bulb went on in my head. It was an amazingly simple revelation. If mercury can shut down the liver's ability to excrete mercury, then this same mercury will slowly accumulate in the liver and eventually poison it, and every other organ it comes into contact with. So the obvious question was, how do I clean out the liver?

Eventually I came across a rather interesting protocol called the *liver flush*. The idea behind it is actually very straightforward. The liver flush is not really a chemical cleaning, but rather a mechanical push. Purge the liver of whatever is clogging its passageways, and you have a filter that can now do its various detoxing and digestive jobs with greater ease and efficiency.

**GLUTATHIONE**

In terms of detoxing, the liver's main job is to produce a chemical called glutathione. This chemical is the human body's master detoxification molecule. While glutathione is produced in every cell of the body, its greatest concentration is found, not surprisingly, in the liver. Glutathione has the ability to grab onto a multitude of toxins, including mercury, bind to it, and carry it out via the feces. It is the human body's most powerful natural chelator, and it performs an incredible number of services for the body in terms of detoxification processes.

Once I understood all of this information, I began to think that the next step to detoxing would be ridiculously easy. All I'd have to do was take glutathione supplements—which I could easily find in any good

DETOX MEMOIR

health-food store—and *wham!* I'd be detoxing my liver and dumping my mercury the easy way. In case you haven't figured it out yet, I really did not want to do the actual liver flush. It seemed kind of…disgusting. To make matters worse, many detox practitioners highly recommended that a liver flush be followed up with an enema. And not just your average, run-of-the-mill warm water enema either. No, I read in several places that the absolute best enema following the liver flush is a coffee enema. I know what you are thinking. I thought the same thing. *A coffee enema? No way…not going to do that…nope…not a chance.* Simply put, the liver flush and the subsequent coffee enema seemed both unnatural and revolting. So I moved on.

Falling prey to something I said I would not do, I went back to the supplements and tried again for a chemical solution rather than choosing the mechanical solution offered by the liver flush. Popping pills was just so much easier than doing all the flushing and enema stuff. I may have lost my health six years ago, but I still had my dignity. Taking supplements would allow me to keep this dignity. Well, I spent a decent amount of time and money taking glutathione and other supplements, but after several months, I concluded I was no better off than I was before…and maybe even a little bit worse. It seemed my glutathione discovery was just another abysmal failure. Another dead end. More wasted money.

I went back into the research. I had missed something along the way, but what was it? After more time spent looking at the research, I came right back to where I'd started concerning glutathione. This small molecule was the human body's main detoxification substance. This had to be the right stuff. Glutathione was too important to ignore. It even had a sulfur atom in it, and I had suspected sulfur was important right from the beginning. So the sulfur was right, and the glutathione was right. It must have been my application that was wrong. Why wasn't my liver's glutathione helping me in my detox efforts? If you do a web search on glutathione + mercury, you will see dozens of studies and research in support of glutathione's ability to take out mercury. But it wasn't helping me as far as I could see. *Why not?*

Eventually, I discovered that the transport vehicle for glutathione coming from the liver is bile. This yellowish fluid is produced by the liver and sent to the gallbladder to be concentrated. In its concentrated form, bile is an extremely powerful chemical that can break down fats, clean up the intestines, and provide a host of other important digestive benefits to the body. Since glutathione is transported in the bile, I reasoned that something must be halting the bile as a transport mechanism. Furthermore, I found out why the glutathione supplement workaround I had tried didn't work at all.

Glutathione cannot be taken orally for benefit. The glutathione molecule cannot survive the harsh acidic environment of the stomach. The stomach's hydrochloric acid breaks apart the glutathione molecule, unless the pill has an enteric coating. But even if the glutathione pill did survive the stomach's acids, it seemed increasingly likely that my bile was not flowing in the amounts that it should be, and I wanted to know why. I needed normal bile flow, and I didn't want to just create a workaround for the problem—I wanted to solve it. Besides this, I began to suspect that glutathione probably works in conjunction with other chemicals present in the bile anyway, so I abandoned the oral glutathione idea completely.

At this point, I made the assumption that my bile was not flowing in the amounts that I needed for good digestive health. This seemed fairly obvious to me at the time. I was toxic, I had food allergies, and I had nutritional absorption issues. These could all be traced back to poor bile flow and the lack of adequate glutathione in my system. I desperately needed glutathione—but how could I get it to where it was needed?

I learned that I could receive glutathione directly into the blood via an IV drip, but this defeated one of my original purposes, which was to find a safe, easy-to-do, inexpensive, and relatively quick detox protocol that I could do myself. Furthermore, a glutathione IV drip was just another elaborate workaround for an obvious problem. I didn't want to just have a workaround, which essentially addresses symptoms. I wanted to attack causes.

CHAPTER 22

# The New Plan

Slowly, I became convinced that mercury had essentially pickled my liver. I was certain glutathione was the main molecule the body creates to clean up toxins. But I knew I wasn't getting the benefit from my liver's glutathione because my health continued to erode as time passed. Since my dental revision, I was no longer ingesting any new mercury on a daily basis, but I felt that I wasn't excreting out the old mercury either. The chelation substances that provided such a huge health benefit to my kids did not seem to be providing me with anything. Obviously something in my detox system was not working the way it should be.

While I was digging into the research, the topic of gallstones kept surfacing. What was the connection between gallstones and the liver? Well, it turns out that gallstones are not from the gallbladder at all. Gallstones come from the liver. Gallstones increase in size and hardness in the gallbladder, but they actually originate in the liver. *Fascinating.* Furthermore, gallstones are just that—they are stones. As such, they represent a significant source of liver congestion. Could gallstones congest the liver and bile passageways to such an extent that the bile and glutathione would never make it to all of the parts of the body where it was needed? This was an interesting question. I didn't know the answer to it, but it seemed to be a very real possibility. I did find out that gallstones are an extremely common problem worldwide. In the United States alone, it is estimated that anywhere from twenty to eighty million Americans have gallstones. Clearly, gallstones are a pervasive problem. I also learned that gallstones are made up--at least in part--of bile salts. *So gallstones are actually liver stones that cause liver congestion. They are comprised of bile constituents—and glutathione travels in the bile.*

Incredible. The big picture started to take shape in my mind with this discovery. I started to see interrelationships where I had never seen them before. Yes, the liver was indeed at the central focus of my problems, because I was mercury toxic, but it was the bile that was the key!

Bile is a liquid produced by the liver and then sent to the gallbladder. Once there, the bile is concentrated tenfold. In its concentrated form, bile becomes a powerful chemical that assists in the digestion of fats. Bile also works to maintain a healthy intestinal acid/alkaline (or pH) balance. In addition to this, bile lubricates and cleans the intestines of toxins, bad bacteria, and fungi as it moves through the system. Obviously, the various roles of bile are extremely important. But what happens when the flow of bile, normally about a half liter a day, is reduced to a mere drip because of a blockage caused by gallstones? Fats are not properly processed, the delicate intestinal pH is disrupted, and because the intestines are not properly lubricated and scrubbed, toxins, bad bacteria, and fungi proliferate. Furthermore, because of the blockage caused by gallstones, glutathione would be severely limited in its ability to detoxify the liver, the gallbladder, the intestines, and perhaps even the pancreas—because again, glutathione travels with the bile, and the bile passes by or through each of these vital organs. The only result that I could see from the long-term presence of gallstones (or more appropriately, liver stones) was that the body would slowly become more and more toxic. The long-term result of this condition would be catastrophic, and it seemed to perfectly match what was happening to me.

Modern medicine states that one of the causes of gallstones is too much cholesterol consumed in the diet. Modern medicine also blames gallstones on obesity and several other conditions. I read much on what the conventional reasons were for gallstones, but frankly, I was not convinced that any of those reasons were entirely correct. At best, they contained only a fraction of the real story. Sadly, I read that unless gallstones are extremely large, patients are frequently told by their doctors that gallstones are essentially harmless. As more research followed, I began to see things differently.

After looking over a great deal of research, I became convinced that gallstones were far from innocuous. Gallstones were tangible evidence that the liver was malfunctioning. The mere presence of gallstones indicated to me that at some critical step, the liver had malfunctioned, and was now producing bile that was unable to remain in a liquid form. This defective bile coagulates into small stones in the many tiny passageways of the liver. Gradually these stones tumble their way to the gallbladder, where they enlarge and solidify over time. This is how gallstones are formed. But why they formed in this way, I had no idea. I did not know why the liver produced defective bile, but it was reasonable to assume that mercury had some role in the process. I felt this was a reasonable assumption because the liver is the body's main detoxification processing station. Most if not all of the toxins that are taken in by the body eventually make their way to the liver. This would of course include mercury. So, even though I had many questions still unanswered, a pattern of sorts started to form in my mind on how this whole dynamic operated. I began to see a type of pathway in this liver-poisoning process. It had taken some time to put all of what I was finding and theorizing together, but the final summation became what I called the Liver Toxicity Cycle.

The Liver Toxicity Cycle, or LTC, is a vicious double cycle in which gallstones are both the cause and the effect of a toxic liver. Theoretically, this cycle was at least one reason for my many strange chemical sensitivities and food allergies. A person with gallstones will slowly become more toxic because the liver-produced glutathione is not present in quantities needed to detoxify that person. So, over time, a person will slowly increase in toxicity until a breaking point occurs. This was my theory, and it certainly fit my own personal history. I had experienced my breaking point approximately seven years ago when I threw out my back, and a huge number of chemical sensitivities started manifesting shortly afterward. In just a few weeks, my health had deteriorated. I had no idea what hit me. All of these health problems just seemed to have come out of nowhere.

# THE NEW PLAN

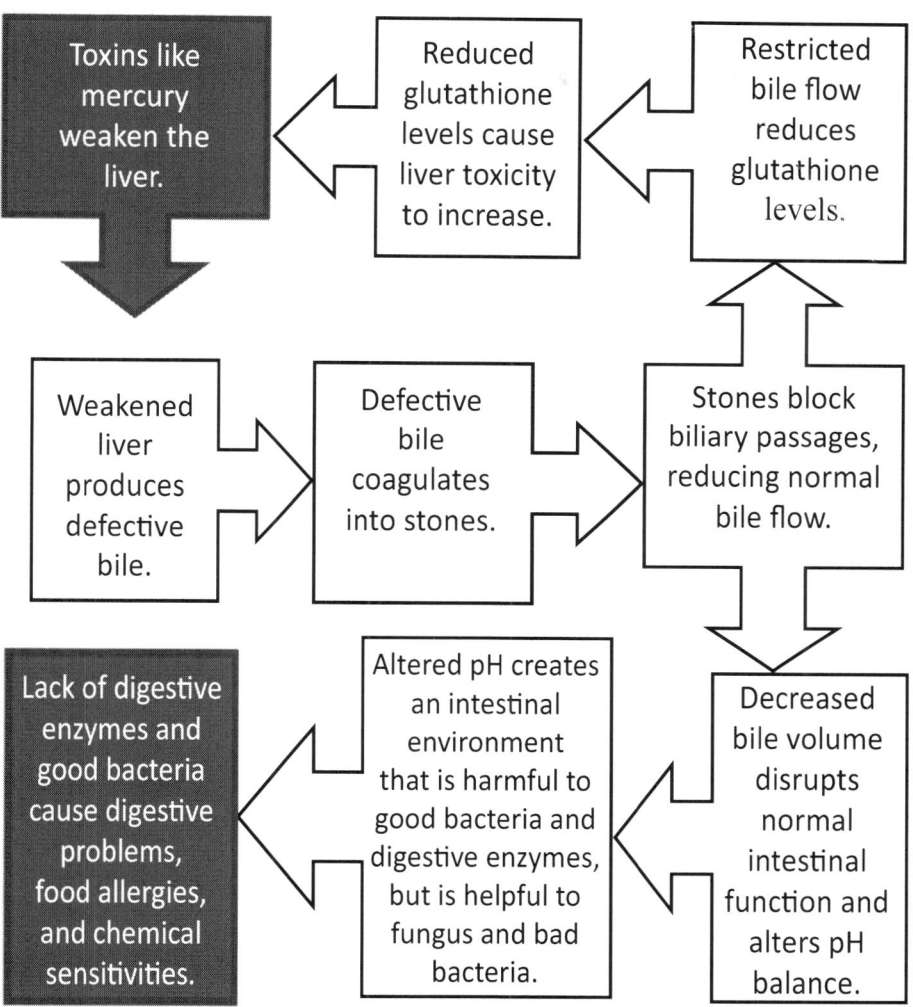

I imagine there are millions of people whose health has collapsed just like mine did, who have thought the very same thing—where did all of these health problems come from? If the LTC was even partially correct, I may have discovered at least a portion of the reason why I was sick, and why so many people like me suddenly get struck with sickness unknown.

The LTC also explained why my kids received tremendous detox benefits from the chelation supplements, while I got virtually no benefit whatsoever. It was the intestinal acid/alkaline (or pH) balance. As a chemistry teacher, I knew that even a very small pH change can have a huge impact on a chemical system. If I did have gallstones, then my bile flow would be reduced, which in turn would significantly impact intestinal pH, which significantly impacts nutrient absorption. I hadn't experienced the same benefits of the supplements that my kids had, because my absorption rates were far lower than theirs. This was due to my unbalanced intestinal pH.

Good bacteria and intestinal enzymes are highly sensitive to pH changes, and their role in maintaining normal digestive operations is critical. Change the pH even a little, and you destroy the enzymes and kill the good bacteria. Food is no longer digested properly, nutrient absorption plummets, chemical sensitivities arise, and it's just a matter of time before serious health problems manifest. This is probably a gross oversimplification of what was actually happening inside my intestines, but then again, I really didn't need to know every detail. I just needed to see the big picture, and it seemed to be the Liver Toxicity Cycle.

> This is probably a gross oversimplification of what was actually happening inside my intestines, but then again, I really didn't need to know every detail.

But, having stated all of this, the LTC was still just a theory. As a matter of fact, I didn't even know if I actually had gallstones. I had neither done a liver flush, nor had I seen a specialist to check for stones. I hadn't done the flush yet because, as I have already stated, the flush just seemed too weird. I didn't see a specialist about checking for gallstones because finding them with an x-ray or ultrasound sounded more like a hit or miss gamble than a science. Gallstones are usually composed primarily of cholesterol and bile salts. This makes finding and viewing gallstones with an x-ray or ultrasound extremely difficult, if not impossible. If this was true for the stones in the gallbladder, which hangs just below the liver, it was even more true for the stones that were deep inside the liver itself. Complicating matters even further, from all I could find in the research, there is no known way for modern medicine to measure bile flow. As was stated earlier, the human body produces about a half a liter of bile a day, but with gallstones, this large volume of fluid would be reduced to an unknown and currently unmeasurable amount.

Stepping back and looking at this whole theory from a macro perspective, I started to see my entire health crisis very differently. I had always suspected that all of my health issues were related, and now I finally had a theory that unified many of the individual pieces. *If you have a mechanism that can shut down bile flow, you have the ability to generate the perfect storm that will ultimately climax with the utter collapse of a person's health.* Perhaps the most diabolical aspect of this whole scenario is that finding the point of origin of this health collapse is nearly impossible. I believe mercury was the point of origin. I was exposed to this toxic metal in large quantities before I was even born. Mercury was behind it all, and yet it again escapes with virtual impunity.

Gallstones also enjoy a measure of "immunity from prosecution" because they do not typically show up on an x-ray or ultrasound. And, for reasons unknown, many professionals in the medical community seem to think that small gallstones are harmless. I thought otherwise. Furthermore, if my LTC theory was even partially correct, it seemed reasonable to assume that it would be only a matter of time before something far worse like colon cancer, pancreatic cancer, diabetes, hypertension, and cirrhosis of the liver would occur. All of these diseases have been linked to the supposedly innocuous gallstone. And once one of these diseases takes hold, no one would even bother with the lowly gallstones, because the disease now presents a much bigger problem at hand.

I knew something about this much bigger problem too, because I had lived through it as a boy. My mother battled Crohn's disease for many years. I had little doubt that this, or some other devastating illness was indeed in my future, unless I figured out how to fix my body.

But all of this was academic theorizing and conjecture. I had done an incredible amount of research into this topic and had thought it through very carefully. It was time to act. There was really only one way to find out if any part of my LTC theory was correct—and that was to do the dreaded liver flush.

CHAPTER 23

# One Very Interesting Year

If my LTC theory was even partially correct, then most toxicity begins and ends with the liver. The liver is the body's main detoxification organ, and since I was seriously toxic, cleaning out the liver would be the first and most important step in the detox process. I wish I could have figured this out seven years earlier. But at least now I was on the right path. I had found an enormous amount of material on the subject of liver flushes. This surprised me. Maybe it shouldn't have, but it did.

In any event, I had done all of the theorizing I could possibly do for the time being. On paper, I seemed to be the perfect candidate for gallstones, but I needed to know for sure. I was still more than just slightly disgusted by the liver flush protocol, but I was also convinced that my theory concerning gallstones and food allergies/chemical sensitivities was correct. It was time to swallow my dignity and just get this thing done.

I was never one to just dip my big toe into the cold water of the swimming pool. When forced to do the unpleasant, I've often found that it's best to run fast, jump high, and dive in headfirst. So I decided that if my first flush was successful—which incidentally meant a toilet bowl full of floating green stones—I would do a liver flush every month for an entire year. Twelve liver flushes in twelve months. *This was going to be one very interesting year.*

If my gallbladder did indeed have stones, some of those stones could have sharp edges. They could also be fairly large—perhaps the width of my pinky finger or larger. Bile ducts are no larger than the width of a standard pencil. *How do you get a big object through a small space?* A good liver-flush protocol should address this very important question. The last thing I wanted was to be rushed to the emergency room because of a clogged bile duct. So the protocol I chose to use for the liver flush was fairly standard and definitely conservative. At last, I was ready to begin.

The entire flush protocol would take fourteen days. For thirteen days, I would drink twelve to sixteen ounces of cloudy (unfiltered) apple juice. This type of apple juice still contains the natural pectin and malic acid, which are thought to be the principal ingredients needed to soften the gallstones. Since the goal is to get a large object through a small space, softening the stones was essential. Thirteen days of drinking a large amount of apple juice didn't bother me, though this was a hefty amount of sugar on a daily basis. Other protocols less conservative than the one I chose called for drinking apple juice for only a week or less. But I wanted to play it safe, so I went with the fourteen-day protocol. On the final day, the protocol called for a fast of sorts. I could eat a 100 percent fat-free breakfast or just fast completely. I chose to fast completely and just drank water and apple juice. After two o'clock, I drank only water until six o'clock. Of course, by this time, I was both tired and hungry but with the end in sight, I pressed on.

Around 7:00 that evening, I drank a glass of apple juice mixed with a tablespoon of magnesium sulfate, otherwise known as Epsom salts. As things of this nature usually do, the concoction of apple juice mixed with magnesium sulfate tasted terrible. But I needed those Epsom salts. They are a laxative and would help clear out the bowels. This is very important. I had read that if your bowels are not clear, you are more prone to vomiting during the procedure, which of course, was something to be avoided. Besides being a laxative, magnesium sulfate also works to expand the bile ducts. This is essential because I was trying to move big objects through small spaces. I repeated the magnesium sulfate and apple juice mixture two hours later at 9:00. I waited two more hours and was ready for the final step. At 11:00, I began the last phase of the liver flush. This was the part that I dreaded the most. I mixed together freshly squeezed lemon juice from three lemons, with a half cup of olive oil. Then I quickly drank it down. Drinking that amount of olive oil mixed with lemon juice was simply awful. But I was determined, and though I nearly gagged, it did go down.

There is a twofold reason behind this oil-lemon juice mixture in the final phase of the protocol. First, drinking pure oil is nasty—plain and simple. Lemon juice definitely increases the palatability of the mixture. Second, lemon juice is highly acidic. Adding a strong acid to the oil means the stomach would not have to act on it much, and it could pass the oil right on through. Once the oil passed through the stomach, the gallbladder would be called upon to empty its bile contents rapidly in order to process all of the olive oil. With the bile ducts dilated (thanks to the Epsom salts), the gallbladder would empty its contents, including any gallstones, into the small intestine. Since the gallbladder had been in a state of fasting for the last twenty-four hours, a strong back pressure existed. Once oil was introduced into the small intestines, the back pressure would finally be alleviated with the release of the gallbladder's bile—and along with this bile, any stones that were in the gallbladder. This was the mechanical push aspect of the liver flush. In a way, the gallbladder would be tricked into violently emptying its contents into the small intestines. The idea seemed logical. But would it work for me?

After I drank the oil/lemon juice mixture, I immediately went to bed. The protocol called for this, and advised that I lay on my right side and try not to move at all. I had to be completely relaxed and motionless so that the gallbladder would start to empty itself. I did just as the protocol said. Exhausted by the lack of food for the day, I quickly fell asleep.

In the morning, I took another dose of Epsom salts at six o'clock and a second dose two hours later. By noon, I was going to the bathroom constantly, and what do you think I saw floating in the toilet? Just like I had seen on the web, there were bright green gallstones floating in the toilet bowl. There were literally hundreds of stones floating right there in front of me. It was a disgustingly hideous and gloriously wonderful sight. It was the sight of

> It was a disgustingly hideous and gloriously wonderful sight.

## DETOX MEMOIR

success. The flush had worked! Over the course of the day, I passed even more stones. It was incredible to think that all of this congestion-causing blockage came from my liver, gallbladder, and bile ducts.

I was astonished beyond measure. And I was also nauseated beyond belief. Passing all of those stones in a very short period of time made me feel like I had just been run over by a truck. I'd been warned about this. A good liver flush relieves pressure, congestion, and pent-up toxins. The flush had broken a dam of sorts, and all of those pent-up toxins were now flowing through my intestines. That's why you frequently feel nauseated immediately after a liver flush. Thankfully, this misery is short-lived. By five or six o'clock that evening, I started to feel like my old self again. The flush was an astounding success. I was able to empty my liver, gallbladder, and bile ducts of hundreds of these bright green gallstones. It was absolutely incredible. I had never seen anything like this before.

Now you may be thinking that these stones are just feces, or even the olive oil itself. I had wondered the same thing. I researched this question and found that others before me had taken their stones into a lab for analysis. Their results were exactly as expected. The stones were a mixture of cholesterol, bile salts, and toxins.

This was the first of twelve liver flushes that I was going to do this year. I thought that one liver flush each month would surely guarantee that my liver and gallbladder would be cleaned up for good.

Well, after a solid year of doing monthly flushes, I found out I was wrong. Instead, at the end of that year, I was still producing generous amounts of pea-sized or larger gallstones with every flush. Either I was doing something terribly wrong, or my body was just incapable of making regular bile anymore. Or there was some other factor preventing normal bile production and flow. Whatever the case was, it seemed clear to me after a year of liver flushes that I was far more toxic than what I had originally thought. I had run out of ideas at this point. But rather than simply doing nothing, I kept doing regular liver flushes, basically whenever I had the time and energy to do so. I continued trying to figure out where and how I had gone wrong. The answers were out there. I just had to find them. And, as was my usual practice, I kept a fairly meticulous journal of all of my data, observations, theories, and new research findings. This journal was very important to me, and much of it became the basis for this memoir.

CHAPTER 24

# The Undiplomatic Breakthrough

I am not a very diplomatic person. I've been told this by friends and family members for years. Even though I've argued this point with them and silently denied it to myself, in the last few years I've come to the conclusion that my friends and family are correct. I'm not diplomatic, and I am not about to start trying to be so now. I have written this memoir in a way that emphasizes facts, with very little regard to the many and varied diplomatic delicacies, which, I suppose, other authors cleverly include in their writings. But really, at the end of the day, my lack of diplomatic skills do not really matter. I wanted to find things that work, and I wanted to record what I went through as accurately as possible. When it was all over, I had made incredible strides to improve my own pitifully frail physical condition. I eventually did regain all those years lost to bad health, and one goal of this memoir is to pass on these health-recovering secrets to you, even if it means sharing information that is crude and decidedly undiplomatic.

I say this as a way of preparing you for the next topic of discussion—solid human waste.

> After well over a dozen liver flushes, I was still producing those ridiculous gallstones.

After well over a dozen liver flushes, I was still producing those ridiculous gallstones with each and every flush. This was strange, but even stranger was the solid waste I was producing during this time. Very often, I would produce feces that had an extremely pungent, offensive, metallic odor. Years ago, I did some work at a local welding shop. My feces sometimes smelled like that old shop. It had an irritating, burnt metal kind of odor. But as strange and irritating as this was, I took it as a very good sign. I felt this meant my body was now purging itself clean; literally dumping the heavy metals that were stored deep in its tissues. I also felt I was eliminating a significant amount of fat too. Fat is an excellent insulator for toxins. If the body cannot excrete a toxin, it often tries to hide the toxin in fat. This dumping of fat was validated with the changes I began to see around my waistline. I hadn't measured my waist, but I knew that something good was happening because my pants were not as tight as they used to be. I wasn't losing weight, really; I was just losing it around my waist. This was good! A very powerful change was occurring, and I felt different. I started to notice that I was getting stronger, physically and mentally. I felt more in tune with my surroundings. These feelings were not just in my mind either. I had hard data to back it.

| POTENTIALLY TOXIC ELEMENTS (17 months) | | | | |
|---|---|---|---|---|
| | RESULT µg/g | RANGE | PERCENTILE 68th | 95th |
| Aluminum | 14.0 | <12.0 | | |
| Antimony | 0.035 | <0.080 | | |
| Arsenic | 0.11 | <0.120 | | |
| Bismuth | 0.047 | <2.0 | | |
| Cadmium | 0.038 | <0.150 | | |
| Lead | 0.52 | <2.0 | | |
| Mercury | 0.07 | <1.10 | | |
| Uranium | 0.11 | <0.060 | | |
| Nickel | 0.26 | <0.40 | | |
| Silver | 0.02 | <0.10 | | |
| Tin | 0.38 | <0.30 | | |
| Titanium | 0.52 | <1.00 | | |
| Total Toxic Representation | | | | |

Shown here is the hair analysis data after approximately seventeen months of faithful liver flushes, chelation supplements, and FIR sauna uses. The improvements were very impressive when compared against the baseline data.

I was certain much of this improvement was due to the liver flushes and their effect on glutathione production. I knew this to be true because my kids and I had done chelation for quite some time. Their hair analysis reports had shown tremendous improvement due to the chelation treatments. My hair analysis reports during the same time period had not shown any real improvement at all. However, once I added the liver flushes to my detox protocol, my lab data greatly improved. The flushes were working, and my body was doing exactly what it was supposed to be doing—eliminating toxic wastes through the organ best suited to accomplish this task—the intestines.

| Toxin | Original Level | After 17 Months | % Increase or Decrease |
|---|---|---|---|
| Aluminum | 25.0 | 14.0 | 44% Decrease |
| Antimony | 0.054 | 0.035 | 35% Decrease |
| Arsenic | 0.11 | 0.11 | No Change |
| Bismuth | 0.040 | 0.047 | 18% Increase |
| Cadmium | 0.029 | 0.038 | 31% Increase |
| Lead | 0.750 | 0.52 | 31% Decrease |
| Mercury | 0.30 | 0.07 | 77% Decrease |
| Uranium | 0.090 | 0.11 | 222% Increase |
| Nickel | 1.10 | 0.26 | 76% Decrease |
| Silver | 0.22 | 0.02 | 91% Decrease |
| Tin | 0.84 | 0.38 | 55% Decrease |
| Titanium | 0.78 | 0.52 | 33% Decrease |

# THE UNDIPLOMATIC BREAKTHROUGH

At least, this is what I thought was happening, because of the numerous times I passed that foul, metallic-smelling, solid waste. It all seemed very logical to me, but it was still just a supposition. I did not gather any quantitative evidence from the solid waste to support this belief. That would have required my collecting a fecal sample and sending it into the lab for a heavy-metal analysis. I just could not coax myself into doing that. Collecting a stool sample is gross. Despite all of those liver flushes and the taking of notes concerning metallic-smelling feces, I couldn't do it. I still had my dignity...sort of.

Here is another breakdown of the data in comparison to my baseline data. Out of the twelve toxic elements found in the hair sample, I saw a significant decrease in the levels of eight elements. While I was extremely pleased with this progress, not everything changing was for the better, at least not on the surface. There were side effects that accompanied these liver flushes, and these side effects were both painful and unpleasant.

Typically after a liver flush, I would feel tremendous for a few days. My lower back in particular would feel amazing. And then, after a week or so, my back would begin to tighten up again. This would increase into a general stiffness that was extremely uncomfortable, particularly during the morning hours. It felt similar to that old lower-back pain I used to have, though not nearly as severe. Also, after a successful liver flush, my face would sometimes have swelling, just like in the past when I ate certain foods. Hives and rashes would also come at times, and the hives would often be very itchy and painful. I also frequently experienced night sweats—the kind you would have with a bad fever. I wasn't sick, but I would often awaken during the night with a shirt that was completely soaked in sweat.

At first I was bewildered by these unpleasant side effects. I was doing something very good in getting rid of the gallstones, and now my body seemed to be in a state of utter rebellion. Where did all of these nasty side effects come from? I was following a strict diet that I did not deviate from, so it couldn't be an allergic response to food. It was almost as if my body was somehow more sensitive to the detoxing process than it had been before. I went back again into the research to try to make some sense out of all of this. Slowly, I found some answers.

Once the gallstones were removed from my liver, gallbladder, and bile ducts, the bile produced in the liver could now flow freely, as it should. All of this newly flowing bile contained glutathione, the human body's main detoxifying molecule. My liver and intestines had been through a virtual bile drought, but now they were once again seeing significant amounts of highly alkaline bile and its powerful detoxifying passenger, glutathione. I became convinced that the liver flushes alongside the chelation had put my entire body into a state of detox overload. In short, my body was detoxifying too quickly for its own good.

I discovered this hyper-detox state is actually an extremely common, even predictable, phenomenon. In fact, it even has a name. It is called the Herxheimer reaction. But through that first year and into the second year of liver flushing, I did not understand any of this. I thought I was either doing something wrong or I was failing to do something right. My Herxheimer reactions (also appropriately known as a healing crisis or a die-off effect) were extremely predictable, and far too annoying to ignore. The reactions seemed to stem from those monthly liver flushes. But I needed to do the flushes because the stones had to be removed. So I was in a bit of a quandary. *If I don't do the flushes, my liver will just increase in congestion. If I do the flushes, I'll suffer those horrible Herxheimer reactions.* But I was convinced that I was on the right track. I had to keep going forward, even if I knew I'd be experiencing Herxheimer reactions, whether big or small. And even though it was embarrassing and unpleasant, the liver flush was a vital key to my detox protocol. I believed it was the main variable contributing to my detoxing success thus far, and I had four reasons for believing this.

First, the liver flush put the liver at the tactical center of the detoxification process, which is where it belongs. The liver is the body's main detoxification and chemical-processing organ. Reducing its congestion by removing thousands of stones allowed the liver and the chelation supplements to do what they were designed to do. You cannot detox yourself with a dirty and congested liver. That was why my kids benefitted greatly from taking chelation supplements, but I did not. I had a dirty and congested liver; they did not. Over the course of seventeen months, I had produced gallstones with each and every flush. Relieving the liver of this much congestion had to make its overall functioning far more efficient. And in this improved state of efficiency, the liver could utilize the chelation supplements properly. Furthermore, in this now uncongested state, the liver would be able to produce bile and the vital detoxing molecule glutathione in the amounts that my body required. The reduction of liver congestion freed up the glutathione so that it could travel throughout the entire intestinal tract, detoxing everything in its path. The liver flush effectively mobilizes the excretion mode best suited for getting rid of toxins—the intestines. Yes, toxins are eliminated through urine and the skin as well, but the intestines are the body's main waste-transport mechanism, and I wanted to work with the natural design of the body, not against it. Because the liver flush facilitated the return of both normal bile and glutathione flow, the intestines could now do what they were designed to do—efficiently get rid of wastes.

Secondly, after most of these flushes, I experienced a Herxheimer reaction. They were fairly predictable. The only other time I had ever experienced a Herxheimer reaction on a regular basis was when I took too many chelation supplements at once. This was an important, albeit painful, discovery. While it is sometimes agonizingly unpleasant, the healing crisis is evidence that a detox protocol is working. The trick was to take the chelating supplements in dosage amounts that were just below the Herxheimer reaction threshold. Once I figured out this dosage amount, I stuck to it faithfully. But the liver flushes put me in an awkward position. I could not dial down the dosage for a liver flush, like I could for the chelation supplements. It was all or nothing. I was getting such fantastic benefits from the flushes, though, that I kept at them anyway, gritting my teeth when the Herxheimer reaction regularly reared its ugly head.

The third reason I felt that the liver flush was the main key to my success was the passage of all of those loathsome gallstones. They came out of my liver, gallbladder, and bile ducts. Gallstones can carry heavy metals. The existence of the stones themselves was evidence that the liver was being detoxed. No, I did not send a bunch of the stones out to a lab to have them analyzed. I didn't need to. Other researchers had done this and had verified that these green stones were, in fact, gallstones and not simply coagulated olive oil from the liver flush protocol. Also, other researchers had analyzed gallstones for their chemical content, and toxic elements were frequently found inside. In my mind, the physical evidence of the efficacy of the liver flush were the stones themselves. They were tangible proof that the liver flushes were effecting some very powerful and positive changes.

Finally, the metallic-smelling solid waste I was producing and the very frequent night sweats were evidence that my body was strong enough to be able to shift into its own self-regulating detoxification mode. Though both unpleasant and uncomfortable, the pungent solid waste and night sweats were further evidence that my body had moved from a weakened state of helplessly and continuously absorbing toxins to a place where it was able to excrete the toxins, which is a great strength.

The only flaw I could see at that time was that I might have been presumptuous in my conclusions. I needed more time to gather more evidence in order to confirm my theories. So after the seventeen-month point, I decided to keep pressing forward with more flushes. I wanted more data, and since I was still producing gallstones, I figured I really didn't have a choice anyway. I couldn't stop now, even if I wanted to. I didn't want to go back to having a congested liver. I really was forced to keep doing the flushes until I could figure out why I still was producing gallstones. I began to suspect that the problem behind the recurring gallstones might be further upstream from the liver. Something was causing the liver to make defective bile that coagulated into stones. What it could be, I had no clue at present. So I kept at the regular monthly liver flushes until I came up with a newer and better idea.

CHAPTER 25

# Fog

In many ways, this is a crazy story. Several times I just had to laugh at the insanity of it all. Gallstones. Metallic-smelling waste. Hives and swelling. Liver flushes. Herxheimer reactions. Night sweats. FIR sauna. So I did laugh, very often. If I didn't laugh, I think I would have just lost it completely. I was an unhealthy mess, and I knew it. But at least I knew I was in a mess, and I knew also that I was slowly climbing out of it. It has been my observation that many, if not most people are toxic, just like me. The problem with them is that they don't even know it. I knew it, and I was making real progress with getting out of it. My own story began with sickness unknown, but my guess is this is many people's story. We're told that at least 15 percent of the US population alone has gallstones. This is a huge number of people, and whether the stones are small or large, they are not as benign as many in the health profession would have us believe. There is no such thing as a benign blockage, particularly in an organ as important as the liver. Gallstones are ticking time bombs. As I was doing all those flushes that first year and on into the second year, I was continually amazed at the sight of the stones. *These came out of my liver and gallbladder. Incredible.*

I would show friends pictures of these stones, in a completely objective and dispassionate state of mind. Most of what I got in response was "man, that is just disgusting." Of course, many of my friends were also thinking "man, *you* are disgusting." While they were usually too polite to actually say this, I perceived from their eyes, body language, and tone of voice that they were thinking this. But I didn't care. After all, I was the one who was dreadfully sick, so I pressed onward despite what the crowd was saying. I had to.

By this time my opinion of the liver flush had completely changed. I was no longer looking at gallstones as disgusting or gross. I now saw them as a huge threat to one's health. They had to put a tremendous amount of stress on the liver. The stones brought inflammation, congestion, and blockage, causing the liver to operate at only a fraction of its normal efficiency. A compromised liver would put stress on conceivably every major system in the body, because the liver has so many important responsibilities.

I also believe the gallstones put added stress on my spine and lower back. I'd suspected for some time that at least some of my lower-back problems were related to the gallstones. After I did a liver flush, particularly during that first year, my lower back would feel amazing. A liver full of stones would be inflamed, making it actually larger in size than it normally should be. This increase in liver size would necessarily put pressure on every other structure in the central body cavity, including the lower spine area. Over time, that pressure on my lower back could lead to a general weakness in the area. Of course, this was just a theory, and I knew I could not prove it. But I knew one thing. My lower back was definitely getting better—much better. It felt strong and flexible, and younger. One day I simply decided it was time to stop wearing the heel lifts in my shoes. I put them all in the garbage and never looked back. I was playing basketball again and doing just about anything I wanted to, athletically speaking. I was still careful not to do any seriously heavy lifting though. I did not want to risk injury doing something foolish. So my days of moving sofas, refrigerators, and other large pieces of furniture for friends and family were now over. But I was perfectly fine with that, and I had an airtight excuse for not doing this type of work anymore. "Uh, you guys better move that piano. I don't want to risk reinjuring my back."

I was making great progress with my detoxing. I was feeling fantastic most of the time, and despite the frequent and annoying Herxheimer reactions, my strength continued to increase. The liver flush truly was an amazingly powerful detoxification protocol. How anyone could call gallstones "benign" was beyond me. Reducing the congestion in my liver had brought me astonishing health benefits. Perhaps even more astonishing was the fact that I had done it with such a simple protocol as the liver flush. Unfortunately, what I thought was a true breakthrough with treating my internal toxicity, most people saw as poop in a bright green disguise.

| | RESULT µg/g | RANGE | PERCENTILE 68th 95th |
|---|---|---|---|
| **POTENTIALLY TOXIC ELEMENTS (26 months)** ||||
| Aluminum | 9.3 | <12.0 | |
| Antimony | 0.017 | <0.080 | |
| Arsenic | 0.11 | <0.120 | |
| Bismuth | 0.050 | <2.0 | |
| Cadmium | 0.014 | <0.150 | |
| Lead | 0.27 | <2.0 | |
| Mercury | <0.03 | <1.10 | |
| Uranium | 0.26 | <0.060 | |
| Nickel | 0.10 | <0.40 | |
| Silver | <0.006 | <0.10 | |
| Tin | 0.05 | <0.30 | |
| Titanium | 0.30 | <1.00 | |
| **Total Toxic Representation** | | | |

I kept moving forward. After approximately twenty-six months from that first liver flush, my journal showed that I had done an astounding thirty-three liver flushes. With each flush, I was able to produce stones. What had I gained from all of this? Well, at this point, I just didn't think or hope I was getting better; I knew it. Shown here are my lab results. I was physically stronger and mentally more alert than I had been in a very long time. It was almost as if I had found a new reality, a wonderfully new and bright one. I realize this sounds strange and perhaps even a bit psychedelic, but I was changing inside for the better. There was no mistaking it. My memory was restored to its former status and maybe even a bit enhanced. My research techniques were increasing in sophistication. I could read scholarly journal articles now and truly comprehend the science that was being discussed. I also started to see my own situation in a different light. I really began to grasp the science of detoxification. I understood it. It made sense. I felt as if my brain had received an upgrade, and I had excellent numbers to back up these feelings of physical and mental improvement.

Here is a numerical comparison of the data, 26 months and thirty-three liver flushes later. The data was impressive. And now, more than ever before, I understood the data. This was another change I experienced. I was able to recognize patterns faster and process complex information far more efficiently. As modestly as I can say this, I felt I was getting *smarter*.

| Toxin | Original Level | After 26 Months | % Increase or Decrease |
|---|---|---|---|
| Aluminum | 25.0 | 9.3 | 63% Decrease |
| Antimony | 0.054 | 0.017 | 69% Decrease |
| Arsenic | 0.11 | 0.11 | No Change |
| Bismuth | 0.040 | 0.050 | 25% Increase |
| Cadmium | 0.029 | 0.014 | 52% Decrease |
| Lead | 0.750 | 0.27 | 64% Decrease |
| Mercury | 0.30 | <0.03 | 90% Decrease |
| Uranium | 0.090 | 0.26 | 188% Increase |
| Nickel | 1.10 | 0.10 | 91% Decrease |
| Silver | 0.22 | <0.006 | 97% Decrease |
| Tin | 0.84 | 0.05 | 94% Decrease |
| Titanium | 0.78 | 0.30 | 62% Decrease |

Now I should quickly add that I highly doubt that detoxing can actually make anyone smarter. I think what was happening to me was that my cognitive functioning was being restored to its normal levels as toxins were being pulled out of my brain. I had no idea how much the heavy metals had dulled my mental faculties until my body was able to start dumping them. The before and after contrast was incredible. I have already mentioned, but have not yet elaborated on one of the worst symptoms of my toxicity: brain fog.

The research on toxicity frequently discusses the problem of brain fog. Maybe it was my vanity, or perhaps it was the brain fog itself, but honestly, I never felt that brain fog was a problem with me. *Brain fog? I don't have any brain fog. My brain is fine. It's the rest of my body that's a mess.* However, all of this changed about a year or so prior to my first liver flush. That was when I realized I couldn't remember the names of many of my students, and that chemical calculations in class were extremely difficult for me to do. This went on for some time. Then I had the revelation. *So this is what they are talking about in the research. This is what brain fog feels like. Ugh. This is terrible!*

The worst part about brain fog was not the incapacitation, at least not for me. People frequently find clever ways to hide or gloss over their mental deficits. Personally, I believe teachers are especially adept at this. And I was no different. This was a strangely ironic situation. I was a chemistry teacher whose body was so chemically toxic that it had created a state of brain fog that nearly prevented me from understanding and teaching the subject of chemistry!

I did not like this new reality, but I felt I could cope with it. But what I could not cope with for long was my shrinking self-confidence. Without a doubt, the absolute worst part about brain fog was the insidious manner in which it undermined my confidence as a teaching professional. I just wasn't

> Brain fog had a subtle way of inducing self-doubt that was downright crippling at times. I felt old. I was becoming mentally feeble—prematurely.

as sure of myself as I once was. Brain fog had a subtle way of inducing self-doubt that was downright crippling at times. I felt old. I was becoming mentally feeble—prematurely. *How can I teach concepts in the natural sciences that I'm not even sure of myself anymore?* I sometimes felt like I was standing still while the whole world just continued to spin on without me.

I had read many times that depression is one of the most common symptoms of mercury toxicity. At the time, I didn't feel depressed, and if someone were to ask me if I was depressed, I'm sure I would have denied it. However, now that the mental haze had lifted, I could see in hindsight that I definitely had been in a state of depression. I just didn't know it at the time. It wasn't until my brain fog finally evaporated that I was really able to see my depression and fog for what they truly were.

Thankfully, that was all in the past. The fog and depression were gone. It had been well over two years since I'd started doing liver flushes in conjunction with the chelation supplements, and I was consistently getting quantitative data that genuinely matched how I was feeling qualitatively. Finally, I was getting the same kind of encouraging data that my kids were receiving as they progressed through their detoxing.

Though I still struggled with the all-too-frequent Herxheimer reactions, I felt stronger both physically and mentally. The quantitative data I was receiving also convinced me that most of my liver toxicity cycle theory was correct. Doing liver flushes and chelation concurrently was a powerful detoxification duo. I was getting tremendous health benefits from this, and these benefits sometimes came in unexpected areas. For example, the white portion of my eyes, the sclera, improved in its whiteness! That was great, and definitely unexpected. I never mentioned this to anyone because it just sounded kind of bizarre. "Hey everybody…look at my eyes. Do you see anything different about them now?" Frankly, by this time, I think that most of my friends and family members were worn out from hearing my latest detoxing theories and results. So I kept the matter to myself and wrote about it in my journal.

Another theory that made it into my journal was a growing suspicion that there might be a connection between clear skin and a clean liver. I never had too much of a problem with acne growing up, but I did have it from time to time as an adult. However, my skin was now very clean and smooth, and I wondered if this also was a result of a liver clear of congestion.

This benefit made some sense as I considered the function of bile and cholesterol. Once the gallstone blockage was removed from the liver's highly intricate network of passageways, the liver would begin to work more efficiently. This included an improved ability to process cholesterol. Bile has direct responsibility over the proper management of cholesterol and fats found in foods. With normal bile flow reestablished, the oils in food would be broken down and absorbed correctly by the body, and excess oils and oily wastes would be eliminated with the bile through the stool—not the skin. Thus I theorized that better skin tone, color, and texture could result from doing several liver flushes.

It seemed reasonable to assume that if bile is not flowing, fats are not properly metabolized and oily wastes are not eliminated properly. But the body has to eliminate the excess oils somehow, so it resorts to a Plan B of sorts, which is to send oily wastes through the blood to the skin for elimination. If the theory was correct, even if it was a gross oversimplification of the biochemical processes at work, then at least some cases of acne were a physical, externally visible demonstration that bile flow was partially obstructed. Does this mean that adult acne indicates the presence of gallstones? Not necessarily. I'm sure there are plenty of other factors at play here, not the least of which would be genetics. I had gallstones galore, but I didn't have a serious acne problem. But I had plenty of friends, young and old, who did have acne, and that puzzled me. As I was working over these ideas in my mind, I began thinking of a friend of mine who had one of the worst cases of acne I had ever seen.

My friend Lance is highly intelligent, ambitious, and he has a great love for the natural sciences. But Lance had a horrible case of cystic acne. I shared my little acne theory with Lance and challenged him to look into the research for himself, which he did. A short while later Lance told me that the connection between clear skin and a clean liver made sense to him, and he was going to try the liver flush. I was cautiously optimistic, because all of this was still very new to me as well. And it was, after all, just a theory. But the science seemed sound and Lance was more than just a little eager to clean up those horrible cysts, so he took the challenge.

Over the next nine months, Lance did nine successful liver flushes. At the end of this time, the results were astonishing. Virtually all of the cysts had either shrank in size or disappeared. It looked almost as if Lance had undergone cosmetic surgery. There were still some scars on his face where the cysts had been, but the change was astounding. Lance was almost glowing with delight. I personally heard many people comment on how good his skin looked. It was an incredible transformation. Perhaps the best part of it all was that most of the people who noticed my friend's amazing new complexion did not know the actual cause of this vast improvement. It was not due to expensive skin supplements with powerful and sometimes dangerous side effects. Neither was a costly surgical procedure involved. Lance and I knew that the credit went to the old-fashioned liver flush, which cost just a few dollars to do, and could be done in the comfort of your own home.

So this was a great victory for my friend. But for me, things just got more confusing. It had been more than two years of doing the regular liver flush, and I was astonished to see that each flush still produced a large amount of stones. *Why was this happening?* I was still missing something in the equation—there had to be at least one other variable in play here that I did not yet understand. I was still a long way off in terms of finding all the answers that I needed to solve this mystery, but the good news was that I was making excellent progress along the way. I had good solid data that things were improving, and after years of discouragement, setbacks, and wrong turns, I knew I was heading in the right direction.

CHAPTER 26

# What Comes Out Goes Around

Several months passed, and I continued to do liver flushes every three or four weeks. While this may seem a bit excessive, every flush produced stones, so I felt that I had little choice in the matter. I continued to research why this might be happening, looking for an unknown variable that was causing this. As I mentioned earlier, I began wondering if something further upstream was to blame. Obviously something was causing my liver to produce defective bile—some other organ malfunction or perhaps a serious vitamin or mineral deficiency. Another possibility I had been considering for some time was the problem of toxin redistribution. The old mercury and other metals present in my body's tissues were liberated by the glutathione surge brought on by the restoration of normal bile volumes. If too many toxins were liberated with too little glutathione to manage these toxins, toxin redistribution was probably inevitable.

Once toxins are freed from cells, the body tries to get rid of the toxins immediately. If this is not possible, the toxins naturally redistribute themselves throughout the body and settle into tissues opportunistically, where they continue their destructive work. In terms of my own experience, this theory made sense because after a liver flush, many of my symptoms—the itchy hives, swelling, the sore lower back, and general uneasiness were noticeably reduced both in frequency and severity. However, after only a few weeks, the symptoms would begin to reappear. When I first noticed this pattern, I simply thought it was time for my monthly flush. I viewed the return of my symptoms as an indication that my body's natural detoxification mechanisms were beginning to get bogged down by the accumulation of trapped toxins. I still think this reasoning was partially correct, but after more research, I concluded it was probably not the whole truth. It seemed very likely that the returning of symptoms at the end of the month was due at least in part to the same old toxins that were being redistributed, and not new toxins that were mobilized by my body's natural detox mechanisms. This diagram may help explain this phenomenon.

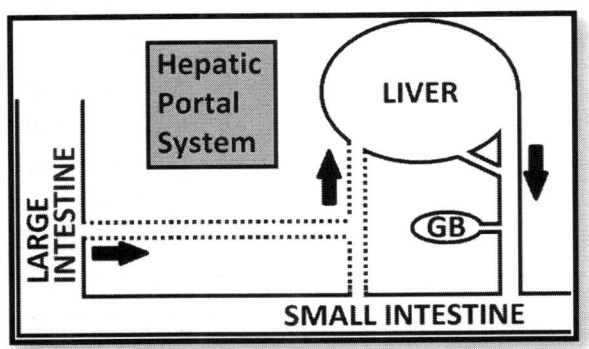

I had no doubt that my liver, gallbladder, and common bile duct were clogged with stones. The regular liver flushes purged these passageways clean, and glutathione rich bile flowed freely into the small intestine for a time. But for some unknown reason, the bile my liver was making was not able to stay in liquid form. It was defective. It coagulated into a semi-solid form which eventually became stones that gradually clogged up the liver, gallbladder, and bile ducts. Because glutathione travels in the bile, it was also dammed up, and the toxins that were moving through the small intestine didn't make it through the entire intestinal system for excretion. Instead, they were picked up by the hepatic portal vein and sent back to the liver for processing.

In all probability, this is what was happening to me. I was having a major toxin recycling and redistribution problem. Many detox experts believe that reabsorption and redistribution of mercury alone can exceed 70 percent! No wonder so many people say that detoxing can be a dangerous business. In a way, detoxing your system is like stirring up the murky bottom of a polluted swamp. It needs to happen in order to clean out the swamp, but you can't do it without clouding the water.

I knew detoxing was essential, and I was definitely getting tremendous benefits from it. However, the recycling and redistribution problem certainly slowed things down for me. But I pressed on anyway since getting rid of some toxins was better than nothing. Even with recycling and redistribution issues, my overall toxin burden seemed to be decreasing over time. I already had evidence of this with my twenty-six-month hair analysis report. I knew my health was improving, but I thought I could do better. So I started looking for ways to cut down on the redistribution and reabsorption of the toxins.

One very easy solution to the problem was simply to increase the frequency of going to the bathroom. Producing more solid waste on a daily basis meant decreased transit time through the intestines, and this would decrease toxic redistribution. Eating greater amounts of raw vegetables was the simple solution for this. I enjoy eating vegetables, and this dietary shift toward raw foods did increase my solid waste production significantly.

However, I found that I could only do this for so long before I got tired of the raw vegetables. It seemed like I was now eating like a goat. *There had to be a better way for a meat-and-potatoes guy like me.*

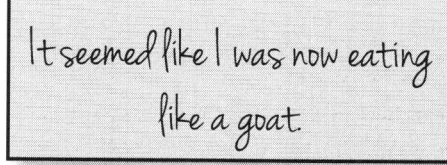

It seemed like I was now eating like a goat.

After talking this over with friends who are far more creative in the kitchen than I am, I discovered the wonders of making a daily juice and vegetable smoothie that tasted fantastic and still vastly increased the amount of waste I produced on a daily basis. This very easy solution gave me the best of both worlds. My body wanted raw fruits and vegetables on a daily basis, and I needed the intestinal transit time reduced. This change would significantly lower toxin redistribution amounts. It was a win-win situation, and I loved the convenience and taste of a delicious smoothie each day. This was an easy solution to a very complex problem.

CHAPTER 27

# Crisis of Healing

Healing takes time. While we all understand this, sometimes our impatience overpowers what we know to be true. This is when we often make mistakes. If what I read was true, for every year that a person has a toxic liver, an entire month of detoxing is required to reverse the liver damage. This doesn't sound too bad until you really look at the numbers of how long you were actually toxic. Suddenly, the healing time starts to look daunting. A twenty-four-year-old person would require *two full years* of detoxing in order to have their liver restored to normal health. No wonder so many people give up on their detox protocols. It just takes too much time.

> A twenty-four-year-old person would require two full years of detoxing in order to have their liver restored to normal health.

Of course, twenty-four months of detoxing for a twenty-four-year-old liver assumes that the toxic individual was actually born toxic. By this point in my journey, I became convinced by the research and from my own experience in detoxing that this was true. That terrifying theoretical leap I had taken was no longer theoretical for me. It was a fact. Toxic mercury from dental fillings, vaccinations, and foods like fish is passed down through the generations in the maternal bloodline. Although I could not prove this experimentally, the circumstantial evidence seemed overwhelming. It was the only conclusion that made sense. The mercury I was currently dealing with came from my mother, my grandmother, and from my own fillings, vaccinations, foods that I had eaten, and from environmental exposure. True, I was no longer regularly introducing new mercury into my system because I no longer had mercury fillings. But I was convinced I was still mercury toxic. I was exposed to mercury at conception. My mercury problem was systemic, with an unknown number of atoms still deeply embedded in my tissues. I had generational mercury toxicity to the second and perhaps even to the third generation.

The good news in all of this was that I was making great progress in my detoxing. Still, I often wondered just how long all of this was going to take. I was now about eight years into my actual detox journey. Naturally, after eight years of dealing with health issues, it's easy to become impatient. Even though the slow improvement that I was currently experiencing told me that my detox protocol was working, I wanted more. But every time I tried to push things faster than what I was normally doing, I would get a good case of hives or swelling or some other symptom that just made me feel horrible. It seemed like it was impossible to go faster with my detoxing because of the constant ricochet effect of the Herxheimer reaction.

The history surrounding the Herxheimer reaction is actually quite interesting. It was also strangely relevant to what I was attempting to do. The Herxheimer reaction got its name from the work of the Herxheimer brothers and their treatment of patients suffering from syphilis. The Herxheimer brothers would inject patients suffering from syphilis with a compound that, ironically enough, contained mercury. They found that if the patients lived through this rather ghoulish treatment, they usually took a turn for the worse before their conditions improved. Their reasoning was simple: the mercury compound killed the spirochete bacterium *Treponema pallidum*, the microorganism that carries syphilis. But the mercury compound could not clean up the dead and dying bacteria, and neither could it clean up the bacteria's waste products, all of which are toxic to humans. These waste products spilled into the human bloodstream and actually caused a worsening of the condition for a short period of time (anywhere from a few hours to a week or more). Hence, the Herxheimer reaction moniker was born.

I believe this phenomenon is one of the main reasons people start a detox program and never finish it. They feel worse in the short term because of the release of heavy metals from the deep recesses of the body, and because of the die off effect of pathogens like bacteria that also might be plaguing the system. This is understandable. People do a detox to get better, not to get worse. They start their detox program, and after a few days they feel terrible. They think they are doing something wrong in their detox protocol. I found this to be true in my own case. I would have a successful flush and feel great for several weeks. But then the symptoms—the hives, the swelling, the brain fog, and the back pain would come creeping back. Other times, I would do a flush in conjunction with some chelators at higher dosages than what I normally took, and my face or feet would swell up after just a few hours. I sometimes felt as if I'd been hit by a truck. At first I had no idea what was going on, but when I found out about the Herxheimer reaction, it all started to make sense.

But there is more to the story. It is not just bad bacteria that dies off when a person is detoxing. Intestinal fungi and other parasites die off as well. The average person's microorganism load is approximately 90 percent good bacteria and 5 percent yeast, both of which provide beneficial services to the body, including nutrient absorption, vitamin synthesis, and powerful immune-system support. The last 5 percent of microorganisms are the pathogens—bad bacteria, viruses, and protozoan parasites.

Look at it this way: good bacteria are like tiny animals that feed on tiny plants, the yeast. After eating these tiny plants and some of the food coming down the intestinal tract, the good bacteria are able to make vitamins and provide digestive services to their human hosts. They also keep the bad bacteria and parasite populations in check, thus rendering invaluable immune system services to humans. When everything is in equilibrium, the system works marvelously well. But the process is heavily dependent upon bile flow, because bile provides the proper environmental pH for these beneficial intestinal microorganisms to thrive. Once you have gallstones, the bile flow goes from a stream to a trickle. A lack of adequate bile flow disrupts the delicate intestinal pH balance. This harms the good bacteria, but it allows the bad bacteria and parasites to flourish. In this bile-deprived environment, pathogens proliferate and excrete their waste products into the human host. The waste products of these pathogens are toxic to humans. Because of the gallstones, bile and glutathione are dammed up. The pathogen's wastes are secreted into the human host in ever-increasing amounts, exhausting the immune system over time. The end result of this condition is an enormous variety of serious diseases.

Some researchers have created a more sophisticated theory surrounding this deranged bacteria growth in the body. It is known as SIBO (small intestinal bacterial overgrowth). The theory goes something like this: ingested heavy metals like mercury quickly begin their destructive work in the human body. The body recognizes this toxic attack as extremely formidable and responds by actually cultivating huge amounts of bacteria and fungi that bind to what may potentially have been a lethal dose of the toxic metal. The bacteria and fungi capture and hold the mercury. This allows the body systems in general and the digestive system in particular to function again, albeit at a diminished level of performance. In essence, the body strikes a bargain. The body accepts the presence and even cultivates conditions so that billions of tiny animals (bacteria) and plants (fungi) can live in the intestines in exchange for their garbage collecting services which sweep up the mercury and other toxins. In this way, even though its heavy metal burden is incredibly high, the body is able to continue operating, though at reduced levels of efficiency. This theory states that many, if not most, chronic infectious diseases that we see today are a result of the pathogenic bacteria and fungi that the body itself is keeping alive.

But this microorganism/toxic metal tradeoff has serious consequences. The harmful bacteria in the intestines produce metabolic wastes that are very destructive to the human body. The same is true for intestinal fungi. In its proper location and populations, intestinal yeast provides food for the intestinal bacteria. But if the yeast overgrows its environment, it can become a raging parasitic tiger. Of particular concern is the yeast Candida Albicans. This particular species of yeast is alive in every human being and can bind large amounts of mercury. In small numbers, the yeast Candida is not a problem. But when the digestive tract loses its normal pH balance due to reduced bile flow, Candida transforms from a yeast into a fungus. It then escapes the intestines and settles opportunistically throughout the body. Candida, as with other harmful intestinal parasites, craves sugar. Of course, just about everyone likes to eat sugary foods, and this compounds the problem. This is one reason why frequent sugar cravings are potential evidence of a system in trouble. People crave sugars because they have a huge number of parasitic mouths to feed. While this may sound revolting, and it is, it gets worse. The metabolic waste products of the Candida fungus and other pathogenic intestinal parasites are dangerous, and sometimes even deadly. These toxins include ethanol, formaldehyde, carbon monoxide, ammonia, and the most powerful one of the group, acetaldehyde.

In this degraded, dysfunctional condition, a person is ripe for a Herxheimer reaction when they begin to detox. For example, after a liver flush, the liver, gall bladder, and bile ducts are now clear. Bile will flow in normal amounts while you are eating a meal. But your body is not used to these levels of bile, even though this level is completely normal. Pathogens like bad bacteria and fungi have been thriving in your digestive system for an unknown period of time. The surge of freshly produced alkaline bile kills massive amounts of the pathogens. Your intestines become loaded with multitudes of these dead pathogens, each spilling its toxic contents into the bloodstream. This causes you to feel absolutely miserable. You have just experienced a Herxheimer reaction.

Far too many times, I experienced hives, brain fog, swelling, night sweats, and just a general malaise after a liver flush. I also experienced these symptoms when I pushed too hard in my detox regimen. At one point in my detoxing, I had hives nearly every morning when I awoke. This happened on and off for the better part of a year! Were these problems caused by the death of intestinal pathogens and their horrid metabolic waste products, or were they due to the chelating of heavy metals too rapidly? I did not know the answer to this question. But I did know that the bright red and itchy hives were constantly making an appearance on my chest, legs, and buttocks. Sometimes the hives would even be on my wrists and fingers. These Herxheimer effects were terribly unpleasant. So I searched diligently for some sort of solution to this constant crisis of healing, but I could not find anything…yet.

CHAPTER 28

# A New Sensitivity

Because we live in a toxic world, detoxing is essential. I was certain this was true. But detoxing can be a painful process. However, looking back, I think that much of the pain I experienced in my detoxing was probably avoidable. But so much of this was uncharted territory for me that I was bound to make mistakes. I kept reminding myself that the good thing in all of this was that cleansing was definitely occurring. The research I found was replete with examples of how the Herxheimer reaction was strong evidence that toxins were on the move. I was getting there. I knew toxins were on the move because my data told me it was, and so did my body. I was feeling better, and really... *different*. That is the best word to describe it. I felt different, as if I was in a new reality. I felt stronger, had more energy, and I was less prone to seasonal sicknesses. I felt much sharper cognitively, and I also had a far greater sensitivity to my environment. This was a good thing most of the time, but not always.

> I felt that I was becoming more in tune with the world around me.

For example, my sinuses had been getting better for some time, and then one day I realized that both of my nostrils were clear, even when I laid down to sleep. This was a very welcome change. I had struggled with sinusitis for so many years. With both nostrils functioning again, I could sleep much more easily and in any position that I wanted. This was great because when the sinusitis first hit me, I could only sleep on my left side. Improved sinuses also meant that my sense of smell was heightened. Suddenly, certain smells that had always been there before started to really bother me. For example, I found that the chlorine smell from a swimming pool was now highly offensive. I used to swim in indoor pools before and hadn't noticed this. But with my new nose, the chlorine odor from an indoor pool or hot tub was almost unbearable. Furthermore, I found the chlorine smell in our own tap water to be quite unpleasant. And taking a shower with this kind of junk water, as I now called it, was irritating. Drinking junk water quickly became pretty much out of the question. The chlorine smell and taste was so bad—I was amazed that I had not noticed it before. I had been drinking junk water most of my life, and now it tasted like it came out of a swimming pool. This had to change. So I shopped around a bit, and then spent about a thousand dollars for a fairly good whole-house filtration system. It filtered out many harmful contaminants, including all of the chlorine and much of the fluoride. It was an expensive upgrade, but I just could not tolerate the chlorine smell or taste any longer. Furthermore, I'd suspected for some time that the chlorine and fluoride were probably not helping my detoxification efforts. They might have even been undermining my efforts. I wasn't sure about this, but reducing my exposure to these harmful chemicals was a welcome change.

Another chemical that I found I could not tolerate any longer was formaldehyde. The smell of formaldehyde now made me sick. This was an interesting problem because I was still teaching high school biology and chemistry. Formaldehyde is practically a staple around the biology lab. *How can a biology teacher not use formaldehyde?* After thinking it over for a time, I came up with a simple solution. I moved all of my dissection labs out of my classroom and into the great outdoors.

So you see, even though my new sensitivity was a very good thing, it did cause some problems, and I had to make some creative changes. But these were necessary changes, because the old status quo was simply no longer acceptable.

Of course, this new sensitivity also affected my detoxing efforts. Even as I was getting more of my life back, I became more susceptible than ever to a healing crisis. The Herxheimer reactions were hitting me harder than ever, and in ways I had not previously seen. Some of the usual detox supplements and even certain vitamins I took now provoked a reaction. The detox supplements that I was taking were good, but I think as my body systems cleared up, these systems became more sensitive to the supplements.

As a result, I had to drop down my dosage amounts of the chelation supplements. This was actually good because that meant spending less money on supplements. Adjustments such as these were needed because my body was working to establish a new equilibrium between the detox protocols and my body's slowly improving state of health. These adjustments were difficult to determine at times, but looking over my journal entries of previous dosage amounts, I was eventually able to figure it out.

I had learned a great deal about how to listen to my body over the past few years. One of the biggest lessons I'd learned was that *little things mattered*. If I ignored the signals, even the small and subtle ones, my body would revolt, and I would pay the price.

As evidence of the new sensitivity that I was now dealing with, here are some excerpts taken from my journal during one fairly typical thirty-day stretch:

- Jan 10th—Have a bit of swelling on my left foot, but feel good.
- Jan 12th—Awoke with a swollen bump on my forehead just above my left eye.
- Jan 28th—Feeling pretty good, but had swelling on the bottoms of both feet today.
- Feb 3rd—Awoke at 3:30 a.m. with a slightly swollen lip. Hive breakout on my lower back.
- Feb 14th—Swelling on the face again. *Happy Valentine's Day*.

So again, this new chemical sensitivity was a good thing, but there were aspects of it that were just a pain in the neck—or face, or foot, or wherever the swelling or hives were found. Obviously I needed some help. I had to find some protocol or supplement that would help reduce these awful Herxheimer effects. Most detox specialists say that the healing crisis is a great signal that the detoxing is working. I agree with this. These specialists also advise people to go low and slow with their protocols and supplements in order to determine the upper limits of their threshold of tolerance. I agree with this too. But frankly, I felt I was already going low and slow enough with my protocols and supplements. What I needed was to find some sort of super sponge to soak up all of the toxins I was releasing, not put the brakes on the progress I was making. It took a little time, but through a strange set of circumstances, I found exactly the toxin super sponge I was looking for. But before I share this information, I need to describe another discovery I made during this time. After this eye-opening experience, I never looked at processed food the same way again.

CHAPTER 29

# Human Canary

My new, heightened level of chemical sensitivity had the unfortunate consequence of increasing the frequency of the Herxheimer reactions. At first I thought this problem would just go away over time. But it didn't. I continued to have very frequent episodes of rashes, swellings, and hives. They were not severe, but they were annoying. Clearly something was wrong. *Am I pushing my detox regimen too hard, or am I eating something that is causing this flare up?* This was a very strange time for me. As I have already indicated, I found that as I progressed through my detoxing, I had to constantly adjust the dosages of some of my supplements. I assumed this was because my liver was healing and therefore becoming more sensitive to the amounts of supplements I was taking. This was very good, but it did require careful monitoring and adjustments over time.

Of course, I also continued to be extremely careful with what I ate. I tried to eat as many whole foods as possible, and when I did eat processed foods, I read the food labels very carefully. I was trying more and more to prepare my own foods, because I found this was the safest way to avoid an allergic reaction. Despite all those cautionary measures, however, unexpected events sometimes occurred.

One day I made a large pot of homemade chili. It was one of my favorite dishes to make, and I ate a few bowls of it. But the next day I awoke with a moderately swollen face. *Argh...not again! How did this happen? What did I do wrong this time?* Extremely upset, I went through the usual checklist of what I'd done, what I had eaten, and what supplements I'd taken. Nothing unusual showed up. Everything seemed to be as it should, except of course, my face. I looked absolutely dreadful—like I'd been in a fistfight and had come out on the losing end of it. After a day or so, the swelling went down, and I went over my steps again to see if I could find where I went wrong. Again, nothing unusual showed up. I was mystified. I had made chili several times before and never had an allergic response. *Maybe my current heightened level of chemical sensitivity had caused the flare-up?* I knew it was the reason for some of my allergic reactions, but I did not think it was the cause this time. Honestly, I was out of ideas. I could not find a single item in the chili's ingredients that was even remotely suspicious. Some time passed, and then I received a call from a friend who knew I was doing a great deal of research on heavy metal toxicity. I will never forget this phone conversation.

"Hey, did you see that story in the *Washington Post* about mercury being in our processed foods now? Yeah…it turns out that some foods with high fructose corn syrup actually contain mercury!"

We talked awhile longer, and I told him I would look into this astonishing claim. The first thing I did was go back to the chili I had made. I checked the labels on all the ingredients one more time. Again, nothing unusual showed up. *Wait a minute! What about the crackers I ate with the chili?* It was a long shot, but it was worth a try. I found the box of crackers and read the ingredients. Sure enough, there it was—high fructose corn syrup.

I did a quick web search and found the article about high fructose corn syrup. My friend was right. In January of 2009, the Washington Post reported on a study that examined the chemical contents of dozens of processed foods with high fructose corn syrup added as a sweetener. Almost half of the foods that contained high fructose corn syrup also contained traces of mercury. This was truly a frightening discovery. Why would food manufacturers allow this?

From all that I could find in the research, materials containing mercury metal are sometimes

> Almost half of the foods that contained high fructose corn syrup also contained traces of mercury.

involved in the production of sodium hydroxide, otherwise known as caustic soda. Well, it turns out this same caustic soda is used in the manufacturing of high fructose corn syrup. I have used sodium hydroxide frequently in my own personal laboratory experiments. At the right concentration, sodium hydroxide is extremely corrosive, and powerful enough to dissolve metal in just a few seconds. I assumed that this is what was happening here—the sodium hydroxide was actually dissolving the mercury metal during the production process. The mercury dissolved by the sodium hydroxide then ends up in the high fructose corn syrup. This is an enormous problem, particularly since high fructose corn syrup is used in the production of thousands of different processed foods, including the crackers I had eaten with my chili.

This was disastrous news. Why weren't more people talking about this? Mercury was in the world's food supply in a form other than seafood! This should have been the biggest story of the year, yet no one I knew was even talking about it. High fructose corn syrup has replaced normal sugar on food labels for over twenty years. The manufactured sweetener is found everywhere. I was astonished, disgusted, and angry. Aside from the insanity of having even more mercury in our foods, I tried to reason it all out in light of what I was personally going through. *Why would I swell up after eating those crackers? I had been eating that brand of crackers for years, and nothing unusual had happened before.* The only conclusion I could come up with was that this swelling was due to my chemically ultra-sensitized state. It was the trace amounts of mercury metal in the crackers that had caused the swelling. In a strange sort of way, I began to see my condition as a human canary as a very good thing. My current detox protocols must have still been mobilizing mercury out of its sundry hiding places, and the mercury was still in my bloodstream in significant amounts. When I ate a food product that contained mercury, because of my chemically ultra-sensitive state, even trace amounts of the metal were sufficient to trigger an allergic reaction. *Incredible.*

The newspaper article did not say that all foods with high fructose corn syrup contained mercury—only some. But how was I to know which foods were tainted with traces of mercury and which foods were not, except by testing each food and waiting to see if I swelled up? This was out of the question! There was no way I was going to do this. Being a canary was one thing, but being a guinea pig was something else entirely, especially with ingesting mercury. I decided that eating any food with high fructose corn syrup was just too risky, and I had no intention of playing around with mercury. High fructose corn syrup was a man-made product anyway, and I had learned from experience that most processed foods are far from healthy. God created food that is good to eat. When man comes along and tries his hand at creating food, sooner or later it seems to end up badly.

This high fructose corn syrup discovery answered many of the stranger mysteries that had baffled me in the past year or so. Many times I had eaten processed foods that I was certain did not contain MSG, but I'd had an allergic reaction anyway. Now I knew why. With high fructose corn syrup now on my radar, things suddenly made much more sense. Chips, breakfast cereal, jams and jellies, soft drinks, bread, cookies, and even my ketchup contained high fructose corn syrup. It was time for another cleaning out of the pantry. Just as I had done with the MSG and natural-flavors products years earlier, I now did with any food product that contained high fructose corn syrup. All of it went into the trash. Again, I was amazed at how much food this was. This man-made sweetener was found in so many food products. How strange that I never noticed this before.

As far as I know, I have only eaten high fructose corn syrup once more since the crackers and chili incident. I had thoroughly researched a particular restaurant's menu items and had found them to be safe for me, except for the ketchup, which did contain high fructose corn syrup. But this was an easy fix. I just brought my own bottle of ketchup. And so occasionally, I would enjoy a cheeseburger and fries from this establishment. Many months after my high fructose discovery, I ordered my usual cheeseburger and fries. After I got home, I noticed the kitchen worker had accidentally put some of their "secret sauce" on my cheeseburger. I hadn't ordered the sauce, but I had eaten it many years ago. I had no reaction to it then. In fact, it was quite delicious. So here I was now, sitting down to eat, and I had a decision to make. I could get up from the table, get on the computer and do some quick research to see what was actually in this sauce, or I could just take a chance.

Well, I was tired, hungry, and my fries were getting cold, so I just ate the meal. The burger and fries were excellent, but eating that burger was a mistake. The next day I awoke with a slightly swollen face. Angry and astonished, I was almost certain it was the sauce. I went to the computer and did the research I should have done the day before. Sure enough, I found that this restaurant chain listed high fructose corn syrup as an ingredient in their creamy secret sauce. I had just discovered the hard way that their sauce had a secret ingredient that no one ever would expect or want.

CHAPTER 30

# An Ancient Remedy

I've always dreamed of living and working overseas in some exotic and remote location. I'm not sure where the dream came from, but it's always been something that has interested me. About this time in my detox journey, I was reading a book by a man who had worked overseas in various remote locations. The author described in great detail how he and his fellow workers used an extremely simple substance to treat snake and spider bites, infections, and a whole host of other ailments, ranging from mild to severe. The simple substance they used was activated charcoal. Whether it was used directly on wounds or bites, or in a poultice, or mixed with water for direct ingestion, the author claimed that activated charcoal was the single best remedy they had for the huge variety of health problems they encountered. After reading how activated charcoal could be used for a large variety of ailments involving toxins, I began to wonder if this extremely simple chemical would be helpful in alleviating the highly annoying Herxheimer reactions that I frequently experienced.

You see, at this point in my journey, I was waking up nearly every day with hives or swelling of some kind. These reactions were not too severe, but they were a constant nuisance and exceedingly embarrassing. I was tired of looking odd, and the constant irritation of itching and scratching had really gotten old. So I decided it was time for another experiment. I had toxins inside of me, and activated charcoal appeared to be an extremely effective toxin antidote. Furthermore, it was ridiculously cheap, and it was, of course, nontoxic in any reasonable amount. I really didn't have anything to lose. Yes, in one sense, this was certainly an off-label use of activated charcoal, but in another sense, it seemed to be right on target.

Whether my hives, rashes, and swellings were caused by toxins being released from fatty tissues or the annoying symptoms were from the die-off effect of bad bacteria and fungi, it didn't really matter. The problem was still the same—toxins were roaming freely inside of me. In order to feel better, I had to neutralize them somehow. The only real drawback that I could find is that activated charcoal tastes like dirt and can make a very messy stain on clothes if you have a spill. But I had a plan for this. Instead of dealing with the activated charcoal in powder form, I purchased activated charcoal in neat and tidy capsules. I was now ready to experiment.

I took a few capsules of activated charcoal one evening and went to sleep. The total amount I took that first night was approximately 600 mg. The next morning I still had my usual Herxheimer reaction, but I thought maybe—just maybe—it was slightly less than the irritation I normally experienced. I repeated the experiment for several days, steadily increasing the dosage. Slowly, I began to see some improvement. After just a few weeks, I was up to 3 or 4 grams of activated charcoal, about a heaping tablespoon. By the time I reached this amount, the swelling and itchy hives no longer appeared at all. I kept that dosage up for about a week and always awoke clean and clear of any rashes, hives, or swelling.

This was amazing! I had found an easy, cheap, and powerfully effective remedy to those awful Herxheimer effects. For well over a year, I had suffered some sort of reaction nearly every day. Now I had gone a full week without any reaction at all, thanks to activated charcoal. After a few weeks of taking a daily dose of activated charcoal, I decided to conduct a test. One evening, I deliberately skipped taking the charcoal. *The hives returned the very next morning.* That was all the evidence I needed. I was convinced. Finally I had a solution to a problem that had nagged me for years. It was an incredible breakthrough.

From all that I found in the research, activated charcoal, which is actually just pure carbon in powder form, is virtually nontoxic in any reasonable amount. The two biggest drawbacks with frequent use is that it binds to metal ions of all types—bad and good alike—and it binds to many if not most types of oral medications. My workaround with the first issue was to take a high quality mineral supplement early in the day. This was not a problem because I was doing that anyway. And just to make sure that the charcoal did not soak up too many valuable minerals, I usually took the charcoal only at night, just before going to bed. The second drawback, charcoal's neutralizing effect on medication, was irrelevant to me because I wasn't taking any medications.

The only other negative I could find in the research was that activated charcoal can sometimes cause constipation. This I personally found to be true. But I had been occasionally taking bile salt supplements and bitter herbs for some time now to make up for what I assumed was a bile deficit because of my recurring gallstones. Bile salt supplements and bitter herbs like Yellow Dock or Dandelion Root have the wonderful ability of increasing bile flow and waste movement, and I found that if I took these daily, they provided all the lubrication I needed to sidestep the constipation issues caused by the charcoal. I was fascinated that such a simple element could have such amazing antitoxin properties.

*How is it possible that a single element could neutralize thousands of different types of poisons? Why carbon? Why not some other important element like iron, calcium, or zinc?* These are good questions, and a little chemistry lesson is needed to answer them.

Consider the carbon atom model shown here. Most forms of carbon have six protons and six neutrons in the nucleus of the atom. Revolving around the nucleus of carbon are two electrons in the first orbit and four electrons in the second orbit. You may recall that it is the electrons that are involved in chemical bonding. The four electrons in the second orbit give carbon the ability to bond to an innumerable

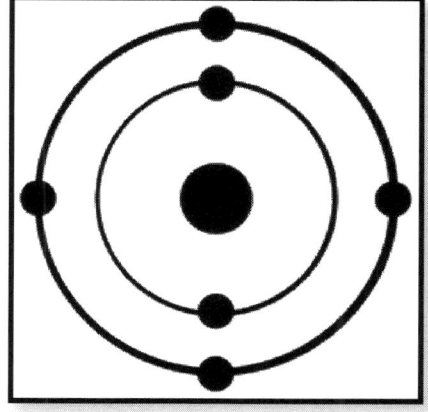

amount of other atoms or molecules. Of all the known elements, only carbon has this unique outer electron configuration in the second orbit. Furthermore, once carbon is treated with oxygen, it becomes activated, and its surface area expands to incredible proportions. It is estimated that a single gram of activated charcoal has the surface area equivalent of a full-sized tennis court! Carbon's ability to bond to a huge number of chemicals and its incredible surface area are the two reasons that activated charcoal is such an effective super sponge for poisons. It can neutralize or at least diminish the damage caused by an enormous number of toxins. Poison control centers know this very well, as do hospitals.

I had actually seen this in action myself many years earlier. When I was an undergraduate student, I worked in the intensive care unit at a local hospital. Activated charcoal was frequently given to victims of poisoning and drug overdose.

When I researched activated charcoal further, I found out that it is actually an ancient poison remedy. Activated charcoal is mentioned in the writings of Hippocrates (circa 400 BC) and Pliny (50 AD) as a powerful antidote for a variety of poisons. The ancient philosophers and historians knew of the incredible medicinal powers of activated charcoal, and they wrote about it for their posterity. But when I dove into the contemporary research on activated charcoal, I was shocked to find that there were very few scholarly studies done concerning this incredible toxin neutralizer. In fact, I barely found anything concerning activated charcoal in the scholarly research at all.

This was a substance capable of neutralizing thousands of different types of poisons, and it was used widely in water and air filtration systems around the world. Despite all this, scholarly studies concerning the use of activated charcoal in the way I was using it were almost nonexistent.

I have heard that the reason for this lack of research into the incredible benefits of taking activated charcoal internally for detoxification purposes is because it is not profitable. Activated charcoal cannot be patented or sold as a prescription, so there is no profit incentive to drive the research. This is a

## AN ANCIENT REMEDY

tragedy. Here was God's gift to a toxic humanity, and it was being virtually ignored in the scholarly research as a detoxing instrument.

Well, I did not ignore the wonderful benefits of activated charcoal. It is an amazing toxin neutralizer, and it was an invaluable deterrent to those horrible Herxheimer reactions. As I looked into the chemistry of activated charcoal even further, I became convinced that it is quite simply the greatest single toxin antidote—anywhere. No other antidote even comes close. Carbon's distinct electron configuration and its ability to assume a form that has an incredibly large surface area is completely unique among the known elements. And activated charcoal is not some rare substance that can only be found in some remote rainforest. Anyone anywhere can create a quick antidote to thousands of different poisons, just by burning some wood, beating the coals into a fine powder, mixing it with water, and drinking it down. What could be easier?

With regards to my personal situation, it is really hard to describe the joy I felt when I saw how effective activated charcoal was at keeping my Herxheimer reactions at bay. No more waking up with hives or swelling. *What sweet relief.* I had finally found rest from the tyranny of the morning. This was the easiest and cheapest remedy I had found yet, and it was about to get even cheaper.

> I finally found rest from the tyranny of the morning.

I found that activated charcoal in pill form was not the most cost-effective way of getting this relief, since I was taking 3 to 4 grams a day. That required taking just too many pills. So I contacted a distributer on the web that specializes in selling high-grade, bulk quantities of activated charcoal. Taking about a tablespoon of the powder mixed in water or juice was all I needed to keep away the highly annoying and irritating swelling and hives.

I know what some of you are thinking. *Eating pure carbon every night can't be good for you, can it?* That's an excellent question. But what was the alternative? The swelling, rashes, and hives I was experiencing almost daily were certainly due to internal toxins. Was having toxins released into my bloodstream all night long with nothing to neutralize them a better option? In my opinion, doing nothing was a far more dangerous choice, and really not a solution at all. Regular skin eruptions and swellings were not only painful and embarrassing, they weren't healthy. I was not certain what the specific causes of the symptoms were, but I was certain that activated charcoal worked to neutralize the cause, and it worked wonderfully well. So, I was committed to slurping down a tablespoon of this element every evening until the Herxheimer reactions went away and never returned. And speaking of slurping, I actually found a great recipe for making my own activated charcoal smoothie. Dissolving activated charcoal in plain warm water makes for a rather gritty drink. I did this for a while, but it always irritated my throat as I swallowed it. Mixing a tablespoon of activated charcoal in equal amounts of hot water and dark cherry juice made for a thick, but good-tasting concoction that I could drink daily with no problems whatsoever. And so, with the activated charcoal now taking care of those nasty Herxheimer effects quite efficiently, another problem was solved, and I moved on to my next challenge.

CHAPTER 31

# The Unexpected Hormonal Connection

Throughout my detox journey, I tried to keep a fairly steady workout routine. I particularly enjoyed lifting weights and running on the treadmill. Sometimes this was difficult to stay faithful to because the malaise and fatigue were simply overwhelming. But when I felt at least semi-normal, I would get into the gym on a regular basis. When I was younger, I'd been fairly serious about bodybuilding and fitness. Just for laughs, a weightlifting buddy and I even auditioned for an old TV show called *American Gladiators*. I made it through a few rounds in the audition but eventually got eliminated, which probably was a blessing because I am fairly certain a few of the guys auditioning for a spot on the show were rolled out of the arena on a stretcher. So, even though my dreams of a gladiator career were permanently vanquished, I have always tried to keep up a regular exercise regimen. It was nothing too serious though—just a few hours a week. But things started to change for me after about the thirtieth liver flush. As I have already mentioned, I was feeling wonderfully different. *Stronger*. Thinking that it might all be in my mind, I simply noted this observation in my journal and kept the matter to myself. But then I started hearing interesting comments from family members and friends that made me reconsider this. My wife was the first to notice. She asked me if I was working out in the gym more than usual because, according to her, I looked "bigger." Another time, after a workout in the gym, a lifting buddy came up to me and said "I know you don't do this, but I have to say, my friend, you looked *juiced*!" (You probably know this, but the word "juiced" in this context is slang for taking steroids and/or growth hormones.)

Well, I told my friend that I definitely was not juiced, but I had been noticing some very good numbers in my regular medical checkups, particularly in the lab results from my bloodwork. I'd also noticed that my testosterone levels were climbing. During my regular physical examination, I had the standard bloodwork done. Most of the time I also requested that my testosterone levels be checked. The reason for this was because several years ago when I had those very serious lower-back problems, I told my doctor that in addition to a horribly painful lower back, I did not have the energy that I used to have. This doctor was the first one to suggest I have my total testosterone level checked. I did as the doctor instructed, and my testosterone level was measured to be a feeble 182. For men, testosterone (or T levels) typically run between 300 and 700, depending on your age and body type.

My doctor said for a person of my age and build, a level of around 300 was probably the bare minimum. He said that a 182 was definitely one reason why I was feeling so run down and tired much of the time. The doctor added that if my T levels dropped to 160 or so, I would actually be in dangerous territory. He strongly recommended that I begin taking testosterone supplements if my levels fell to that point. I did not want to go down the road of hormonal supplements, and I told the doctor this directly. He agreed that it wasn't the best course of action, but should my levels fall by another twenty points, he felt there was no other safe alternative. I had no desire to take testosterone supplements. I kept thinking that there had to be a better way—a more natural way.

It wasn't too long after this conversation that I began my monthly liver flushes. After about fifteen months of doing the flushes, I had more bloodwork done. I was particularly interested in my T levels. After a year and a half of regular liver flushes, my testosterone levels had climbed from the paltry 182 to a semi-normal 283. That was a 55 percent increase, and I was doing it the all-natural way. Greatly encouraged by this improvement,

I kept at it. About six months later, I was tested again and it came back at a respectable 306. That's a 68 percent increase from my baseline data.

I believe the monthly liver flushes worked in conjunction with the chelation supplements to achieve this impressive improvement, and not simply the supplements or the flushes alone. I have three reasons to support this belief. First, I had been taking supplements by the handfuls for several years prior to the liver flushes, and my T levels were either stagnant or steadily going down. I know this because in those early years, I was gradually becoming weaker and more fatigued. Back in those days, general malaise was the order of the day for me. I just didn't have much energy most of the time, and I didn't know why. I was tired and weak, and my lethargy was, at times, palpable. Testosterone was not even on my radar until my doctor suggested I have it tested. So it was obvious that the supplements I was taking certainly weren't affecting my T levels in a positive way.

The second reason I think the liver flush and chelation supplement combination worked in a powerful and possibly synergistic manner to improve my T levels is because of testosterone's relationship to another hormone—cortisol. My theory for this is very simple. My body was under a tremendous toxic burden, and this caused a great deal of stress to a variety of body systems. Cortisol is a hormone produced by the adrenal glands in response to, and to counteract, stress. If I understood the research correctly, when the body produces a great deal of cortisol, it produces only scant amounts of testosterone. The relationship between cortisol production and testosterone production is an inverse one. As I did those monthly liver flushes while simultaneously taking chelation supplements, I was relieving my body of a massive toxic burden. This greatly reduced the stress levels on my system, which in turn reduced my body's need for high levels of cortisol. As cortisol production decreased, my testosterone levels increased, and I went from 182 to 283 to 306 over a two-year period. I kept it going for another few years, and eventually my T levels maxed out at a rather beastly 512. *Amazing*. This was a whopping 181 percent increase, and it was done without any hormone supplementation.

The third reason I felt the liver flush and chelation supplements worked to improve my T levels has to do directly with mercury itself. From all I could see in the research, mercury also has a powerful relationship with testosterone. Apparently, the human body in general, and the male human body in particular, cannot tolerate high levels of mercury and testosterone simultaneously. For some reason, which I confess I do not fully understand, testosterone greatly exacerbates the deleterious effects of mercury on the human system. I theorized that perhaps the body deliberately lowers its testosterone production in order to avoid these effects. After more than a year of taking chelating supplements alongside monthly liver flushes, I assumed that my overall mercury burden was reduced to a point where my body could begin to restore testosterone back to its normal levels. Again, this was all just a theory that I had gleaned from the research, but it made sense to me, and it certainly applied to my situation quite accurately.

Maybe it's the ex-bodybuilder in me, but I think this memoir would be incomplete unless I give the readers out there—especially the guys—some honest and friendly advice about boosting hormonal levels. If you are actively involved in health and fitness, doubtless you have heard and read something about this topic. I think it is safe to say that much of what you have heard about boosted testosterone levels is probably true. I had heard the same things. Now I actually experienced it.

> Much of what you have heard about boosted testosterone levels is probably true.

Boosting testosterone levels allows anybody interested in bodybuilding to get big—really big. After my T levels passed into the 300 range, I got back into the gym a little more frequently than I had before. I did this because, for one, I actually had the energy to lift weights more frequently, and two, because I was curious to see how far I could take this thing. I bulked up far more easily and faster than I ever could have done, even a decade earlier. Of course, this was just my personal experience. I did not do any actual testing and measuring or any sort of experiment. I just tried to make some overall observations and general comparisons between the old me and the new me. From all I could see, the new me was a greatly improved model.

Elevated T-levels increased my endurance and made me less prone to injury, which is a big plus for anyone, especially athletes. My overall mood was vastly improved, and I even began to sleep better. This really came in handy because I was now a science teacher by day and a graduate student by night. I didn't get a whole lot of sleep during those years, but I was doing fairly well with it. And if I needed a little shut-eye, I found that a fifteen-minute nap in the afternoon was all that was required to keep me going well into the night. A rapidly elevated testosterone level provided incredible life benefits. Believe me when I say this: when you go from a testosterone level of 182 to 512 over a relatively short period of time, you look, feel, and think very differently.

I never took any form of hormonal supplements back when I was into bodybuilding, but I had seen old syringes in the locker room garbage can. Now I understood why they were there. Athletes are competitors. They are always looking for an advantage. Boosted T levels give you a huge advantage. Plus, the rush of energy, stamina, strength, and overall good feeling you get with a high T level is totally awesome. On a moral level, I began to see testosterone as an amplifier of sorts. If your heart and mind are right, I believe boosted T levels can make you a much better person. But if your heart and mind are wrong, I have no doubt that boosted T levels will make you worse. And not just a little worse, particularly in the area of your sexuality. I had heard how powerful hormonal increases are, and now I truly understood it. Hormonal increases are dominant. They are life changing. But most importantly, they should never be trifled with.

CHAPTER 32

# Convergence

Although I was now making excellent progress, I still had many questions and several perplexing problems to solve. The main problem I was still facing was the recurring gallstone issue. I had seen fantastic improvement in my hair analysis data. My immune system was far stronger, and the Herxheimer reactions were mostly under control. My energy levels were terrific, my testosterone level had more than doubled, and my lower back felt fantastic. I was convinced that my liver toxicity cycle theory was correct as far as it went, but the evidence now seemed to indicate that the theory was incomplete. Something was missing. It seemed reasonable to assume that a toxic liver would produce defective bile and a clean liver would not. Of course, I had no actual proof that my liver was clean, but this seemed like a safe assumption after all of those liver flushes. But I was still producing those ridiculous gallstones! *A clean liver will produce gallstones? That doesn't sound right. What was I not seeing here?*

Because my testosterone levels had improved so dramatically—and I assumed my cortisol production had, in turn, returned to normal levels—I started to wonder if maybe there were other hormone levels that were either irregularly elevated or suppressed due to my toxicity. Hormones are astounding chemicals that profoundly impact the human system. Only a very small amount of a particular hormone is needed to effect huge changes. *Could it be possible that my gallstone issue was somehow related to hormones?* At first glance this thought seemed like a stretch—a really big stretch. But then again, I seemed to have established a connection between liver flushes, cortisol, and testosterone, so I felt that a gallstone–hormone connection was at least possible. I knew for certain that my body chemistry was still unbalanced, because I still had strong chemical sensitivities. I did not know if I had gotten all of the mercury out, but I did know that hormones are chemicals that are extremely sensitive to toxic elements like mercury.

And so with these clues and a fair amount of scientific speculation, I dove into the research looking for connections. To my utter astonishment, in a very short period of time I found a sizable amount of information linking gallstones to thyroid hormones. It was a shocking discovery. I also found information linking mercury toxicity to thyroid hormone irregularities. In short, even though I had significant doubts at first, I found ample evidence that suggested a strong connection between mercury, gallstones, and hormones. Mercury toxicity, thyroid functioning, hormone production, and gallstones all appeared to be strongly related. What I had originally thought were several unrelated ideas were now conjoined under a single umbrella. From these ideas and from the research that followed, I created another theory—my theory of convergence.

Very early on in my detox journey, I had a feeling that the element sulfur was somehow powerfully involved in this toxic mess that I was in. But I didn't know how or why. I did find that taking MSM (methylsulfonylmethane) made me feel better, and I knew that the body's central detoxing agent, glutathione, also contains sulfur. So it seemed reasonable to assume that my toxicity somehow had created a sulfur deficiency, and MSM helped to relieve this deficiency. Sulfur is found throughout the body in enzymes and proteins, and mercury is able to disable both proteins and enzymes because of its strong attraction to sulfur. But sulfur is in the same family as selenium, an element that is intricately involved in thyroid hormone production. Sulfur and selenium are in the same column on the periodic table. Chemicals in the same column on the table share many common characteristics.

With this in mind, I assumed that mercury would have a similar attraction for selenium as it does for sulfur. After only a little digging, I not only found plenty of research to validate this assumption, I found that mercury actually has a *greater* affinity for selenium than it does for sulfur! This was an extremely important discovery, because it showed me that the thyroid is particularly vulnerable to the ravages of mercury because the thyroid contains a huge supply of selenium. *Another piece of the mystery was coming together.* Now I needed to see if there was a link between selenium and gallstones. After only a small amount of research, I found that there are actually several connections between selenium and gallstones. And not surprisingly, hormones are involved in the middle of it all.

| Triiodothyronine | Thyroxine |
|---|---|
| $C_{15}H_{12}I_3NO_4$ | $C_{15}H_{11}I_4NO_4$ |

Everyone needs selenium. You don't have to look too far to discover that the thyroid gland uses a tremendous amount of selenium to process the vital hormone triiodothyronine, or T3, from its source molecule thyroxine, or T4. These hormones affect pretty much every area of the body: metabolism, temperature, heart rate, growth, reproduction, and much more. Obviously, the T3 and T4 thyroid hormones are extremely important. Triiodothyronine is a mouthful for sure, but this big name tells you quite a bit about the molecule: "Tri" means three; "Iodo" stands for iodine; "Thy" refers to the thyroid; and "Ronine" refers to tyrosine, the base amino acid used in the construction of both T3 and T4. So, triiodothyronine is a molecule that contains three iodine atoms and is generated by the thyroid gland. T4, or thyroxine, is another thyroid hormone that contains four iodine atoms. Think of thyroxine as the raw material or building block for triiodothyronine because T3 is built from T4.

This background information on thyroid hormones is fairly important, because as I was doing research into my theory of convergence, I found some very interesting facts concerning toxicity and thyroid hormones, including the following:

A. Selenium is required for the conversion of T4 into T3, and since mercury has a strong affinity for selenium, mercury can and will disrupt the T4 to T3 conversion process.

B. The entire human blood supply passes through the thyroid gland on an almost hourly basis. Therefore, blood that contains traces of mercury will have easy access to the thyroid's selenium-rich hormone receptor sites, reducing the thyroid's ability to make hormones.
C. Most of the T4 to T3 conversion occurs in the liver and the intestines—not the thyroid. Mercury has been shown to damage all three areas—the intestines, the liver, and the thyroid, so mercury can shut down thyroid hormone production in areas other than the thyroid gland itself. This was particularly important to know, because it told me that even if my thyroid checked out fine with the lab, my thyroid *hormones* could still be unbalanced.
D. T4, or thyroxine, is strongly involved in metabolism, including the metabolism of cholesterol that occurs in the liver.

From all of this data, it was plain to see that mercury can seriously impair not only the thyroid gland, but it can also disrupt the activity of both T3 and T4, found and produced elsewhere in the body. While this was all very important to consider, my focus was still on looking for a link between hormones and gallstones. This is why the last point caught my eye. "T4, or thyroxine, is strongly involved in metabolism, including the metabolism of cholesterol that occurs in the liver." *Thyroxine is vital for the processing of cholesterol in the liver. But…the main component of gallstones is cholesterol. Hmm. I wonder if that's the connection.*

It took just a few minutes to find studies that linked thyroxine deprivation to gallstones. I had just found another huge missing piece to the puzzle. *Thyroid hormonal imbalances are linked to gallstone formation.* This was an absolutely incredible discovery. This is why a clean liver can still make gallstones, because the problem is outside of the liver. The problem was thyroid hormone production, and this problem, I presumed, was due to toxicity.

But there was even more. Let's review again some of the basics for just a moment. The liver produces bile—about half a liter a day—and sends it to the gallbladder, where it is concentrated tenfold. When fat is consumed in the diet, it travels through the stomach and into the small intestine. The body senses the presence of fat, and causes bile to be released from the gallbladder to process this fat. The bile travels down the common bile duct and into the small intestine. There is a small circular muscle at the point where the bile duct intersects with the small intestine. This muscle is known as the sphincter of Oddi. This sphincter muscle has an extremely important function. It acts as a release valve for both bile and pancreatic juices. If the sphincter of Oddi is working properly, both bile and pancreatic juices will flow into the small intestine at the proper times and in their proper amounts. But if this muscle is damaged or malfunctioning, both bile and pancreatic juice will experience a backup. This was all very interesting, but it did not seem to connect with what I was looking for until I found this simple fact hidden in the research: the sphincter of Oddi has thyroxine hormone receptor sites!

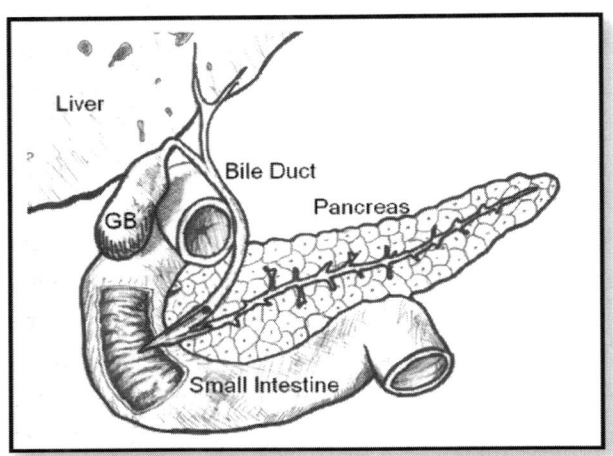

There it was again—another connection between the thyroid and gallstone formation. As far as I could see from the research, the sphincter of Oddi receptor sites and the thyroxine hormone act in a type of lock-and-key relationship, with the hormone being the key to open the sphincter lock. If not enough thyroxine is available, the lock stays shut more often than it should, which effectively causes both the bile and pancreatic juices to experience a backup. Since thyroxine also controls cholesterol metabolism, I assumed this affected bile consistency. Have you ever tried to pour hot bacon grease down the kitchen sink drain? It doesn't flow very far. It cools rather quickly, and then it just sticks to the pipes. This is what appears to happen with a thyroxine deficiency and normal bile flow. And, because of a lack of thyroxine, the sphincter of Oddi is shut anyway. There is no place for the sludge-like bile to go, so the bile just coagulates into gallstones. From all I could see in the research, I was now convinced that thyroid hormonal imbalances lead to gallstones.

Yes, my theory of convergence was just that—a theory. But if it was correct, I imagined there could be an incredible number of health-recovering discoveries that could result from an extension of this theory. Just think about the number of people with gallstone problems who are also taking cholesterol medication! And what about people with diabetes or even pancreatic cancer? Since thyroxine is directly involved in the operation of the sphincter of Oddi, and this sphincter muscle controls the release of pancreatic juices, there was now a connection between toxicity and thyroid disease, diabetes, and even pancreatic cancer. Because the sphincter isn't working properly, pancreatic juices just sit there at the intersection of the small intestine, held up by the sphincter of Oddi's stoplight. The bile is also held up by this stoplight, but bile is different from pancreatic juices. Bile is far more resilient, and because of its high cholesterol content, over time it simply coagulates into stones. That's not good, but it is far preferable to what happens to pancreatic secretions. Pancreatic juices are loaded with important enzymes. Unlike bile, enzymes are notoriously sensitive to pH changes, temperature changes, and time. They denature over time and eventually putrefy. Coagulation on one hand, putrefaction on the other. While both are bad, I preferred coagulation. Putrefaction of pancreatic juices sounded like a precursor to cancer to me.

This theory of convergence opened up a whole new world of ideas, problems, and possible solutions right before my eyes. I wanted to dig further into this theory, but I had to keep my focus on what I was looking for in the first place. I was looking for the reason for my own recurring gallstone problem. And I think I had just found it. The gallstone problem did in fact originate outside of the liver. It began with a thyroid hormone problem. *Cleaning out the liver is not enough. I need to clean out my thyroid gland as well. If I can do this, the gallstone problem should go away.*

Was this the last word on this very complex connection? Certainly not. Actually, what I really had here was not much more than a fairly well-substantiated array of interconnected ideas. But I was moving forward anyway. Time was critical, and I had to solve the problems that I was facing as soon as possible. So, at this point in my investigation, I made several key assumptions that would guide my steps as I moved forward.

> Cleaning out the liver is not enough. I need to clean out my thyroid gland as well.

First, I assumed that my thyroid was polluted with mercury and needed to be cleaned. Secondly, even though mercury could disable thyroxine production outside of the thyroid gland (in the liver and in the intestines), I assumed that this problem was already solved. Mercury in the liver had probably been eliminated due to all of those successful liver flushes. And, I assumed that glutathione-rich bile flowing through the intestines had cleaned up the mercury in the intestines. Of course, I could have been wrong about these assumptions. But for the time being, I was moving forward as if these assumptions were correct. As unscientific as this sounds, this just felt like the right thing to do.

If I was able to clean my thyroid successfully, the evidence would be in subsequent liver flushes. If I did a flush that did not produce the abundance of stones I was accustomed to seeing, I could assume that my body was now producing thyroxine in sufficient amounts. These higher levels of thyroxine should fix the cholesterol metabolism problem in the liver and open the sphincter of Oddi at the right times. This should eliminate or seriously reduce the gallstone numbers.

While I liked my theory of convergence, it was still just that—a theory. I needed to test it. I began researching how exactly I could clean out and reboot a toxic thyroid. In a fairly short period of time, I put together a plan on how to do this. Beyond the results I was hoping for, a newly rebooted thyroid would have many other health benefits as well, not the least of which would be a boost in my metabolism. That, of course, sounded fantastic. Everyone wants a boosted metabolism.

The science all made sense to me. And, at least on paper, it all seemed to be converging quite nicely. Things were really looking great with this new plan, but now it was time to test it, to see if it actually worked.

CHAPTER 33

# Thyroid Reboot

The more I researched the connection between mercury and the thyroid and how it was linked to gallstones, the more I liked my theory. Convergence had definitely occurred for me. *Finally, after approximately nine years of struggling with all of these strange and crippling health problems, it all seemed to be coming together.* And my thyroid reboot protocol was shaping up nicely as well. From all that I could find in the research, there was no flush that existed to clean up a toxic thyroid like there was for the liver. But I was completely fine with this, because I was pretty tired of the flushing thing anyway. I found that cleaning up a polluted thyroid could be done using supplements. Yes, it was back to taking supplements, but this time, I was aiming at a specific target. I planned to clean up and reboot my thyroid with just a few key supplements, which I simply called my *thyroid boosters*.

> Yes, it was back to taking supplements, but this time, I was aiming at a specific target.

Of course, taking a high quality multivitamin was an essential part of any detox protocol. I had known this for years and had been doing it for a long time, but my thyroid hormones were obviously still messed up. From all I could find in the research, there were three steps in the chain of command on thyroid hormone production: the brain (hypothalamus and pituitary), the thyroid gland, and thyroid hormone production in the liver and intestines. This was the chain of command, and my thyroid boosters would be intricately involved in each part of this chain.

The first part was the brain-thyroid connection. The key element here is zinc. This silvery metal has a role in the creation of hormones upstream from the thyroid gland. The brain produces hormones that tell the thyroid what to do, and the thyroid produces hormones that tell the body what to do. Zinc is a key element in this first step, so I increased my current supplemental intake of zinc to 40 mg per day. This amount seemed sufficient to support the first step. The second of my three thyroid boosters was the element selenium. I knew selenium was an important thyroid booster, because it controls the thyroxine (T4) to triiodothyronine (T3) conversion, both in the thyroid gland and elsewhere in the body. Selenium is also highly vulnerable to mercury's influence because of its affinity for this element, so I made sure that I had plenty of selenium on a daily basis. From my research, 200 mcg of selenium daily would be sufficient for my needs. The final thyroid booster was iodine. It was obvious that iodine had to be a key booster, because at least half of the T3 and T4 molecules were made up of iodine. Iodine was also known to protect the body against the destructive influences of mercury, so I made sure that my iodine intake was also more than sufficient. But here is the weird thing—I had *already* been taking zinc, selenium, and iodine at their recommended dietary allowance (RDA) amounts for several years. Still, the evidence before me strongly suggested that I was not making enough thyroid hormones because of the existence of those recurring gallstones.

So I focused most of my attention on this third element in the thyroid boosters—iodine. As I really dug into the research, I started to think that I had been falling prey to what chemists call the "limiting reagent." In chemistry, a limiting reagent is the one key ingredient needed for a chemical reaction to occur. That single key ingredient has a tendency to be in very short supply, and because of that, it essentially drives the entire chemical reaction. Or limits it. All of the other elements found in thyroid hormones seemed abundant in supply, except iodine.

| Triiodothyronine | Thyroxine |
|---|---|
| $C_{15}H_{12}I_3NO_4$ | $C_{15}H_{11}I_4NO_4$ |

As has already been discussed, thyroid hormones contain huge amounts of iodine. Here again are the two main thyroid hormones. The elements in both hormones are the same, but in differing amounts. T3 and T4 both contain carbon, hydrogen, nitrogen, oxygen, and of course, iodine. There was no way that carbon or any of those other elements were my limiting reagent. Those elements are found in everything. The only thing that made sense was that iodine was the limiting reagent. *Iodine was holding back my normal thyroid hormone production.* No other conclusion made sense.

Of course, I had no way of knowing this for sure, but the chemistry appeared sound. Thyroxine alone is 65 percent iodine, so it seemed reasonable that I would need large amounts of iodine in my diet in order to build thyroid hormones. But exactly how much iodine would I need? I was certain I was getting well over the RDA amounts of iodine. It was in my daily multivitamin, in my foods, and even in iodized salt. I estimated my current intake of iodine with diet, supplements, and iodized salt to be roughly 500 mcg per day. On the surface, it seemed that this should have been enough iodine. Evidently it wasn't. Assuming my reasoning was correct, if my current iodine intake was truly sufficient, my thyroid hormone problem would have spontaneously resolved itself years ago. Obviously that did not happen.

The only rational conclusion was that iodine was indeed the limiting reagent, and I needed a great deal more iodine than what I was currently taking. I needed to create an entirely new environment in my system that was much more favorable toward constructing generous amounts of T3 and T4 hormones. These notions concerning iodine were only strengthened when I found research stating that iodine could be used to clean up the mercury sitting on the thyroid hormone receptor sites. *Iodine is a mercury chelator? Amazing!* This was an important discovery, because I speculated that mercury, because of its attraction to selenium, was sitting on these hormone receptor sites. It appeared that iodine was both a builder of hormones and a cleaner of toxins. This was a huge revelation.

If the research was correct, and at this point I was not even close to being certain that it was, I needed to increase my iodine intake perhaps a hundredfold! In order to clear away the mercury from thyroid hormone receptor sites and to provide the essential raw material for the T3 and T4 hormones, I needed to slowly increase my current 500 mcg iodine daily intake to an incredible 50 mg per day. *Fifty mg of iodine a day? That doesn't sound healthy—it might even be dangerous.*

I saw this question frequently in the research, but I also found the remedy for this in the research as well. The key for a large iodine intake was the other two thyroid boosters, along with a good multivitamin. If selenium, zinc, and the other nutrients were in abundant supply, selenium-based enzymes would closely monitor the T4 to T3 conversion process so that my thyroid remained in balance. The key to maintaining this balance were high quality selenium and zinc supplements. From all I could find in the research, this was absolutely essential in order to keep the thyroid from slipping into an overacting (hyperthyroidism) or underachieving (hypothyroidism) pattern.

Of course, there was another way. There always is. I could choose the synthetic route. I had found research in support of taking synthetic thyroxine supplements to get rid of gallstones. But I didn't want to use this workaround for a variety of reasons. First, simply taking thyroxine supplements would still leave me with a tired and polluted thyroid. I wanted to clean up the mercury mess, not step around it. Furthermore synthetic thyroxine required a prescription, and that was something I didn't want to do. I wanted something bigger. Something better. I wanted to clean up and reboot the thyroid naturally, and I was going to use my thyroid boosters to do it.

The increased amount of iodine would clear away some of the mercury atoms stubbornly sitting on the thyroid hormone receptor sites, which should boost thyroxine production dramatically. Some of this newly generated thyroxine would go to the liver, in order to assist in cholesterol metabolism, thereby reducing bile coagulation. Another portion of this newly manufactured thyroxine would go to the bile duct–small intestine interface, where it would provide the essential key to open the lock on the sphincter of Oddi at the proper times. If it all worked according to plan, this thyroid reboot would result in either the complete elimination of gallstones, or a serious reduction in their numbers and sizes. My theory seemed legitimate, but I still had some doubts.

According to my journal, the next liver flush was number forty. I had done thirty-nine liver flushes and was still producing gallstones. *And I thought way back when I first started this journey that six or seven flushes would probably be enough to get my liver clean and clear. How wrong I was.* At least now, assuming the thyroid reboot theory was correct, I knew why that estimation was wrong.

According to my journal, the last three flushes had been extremely productive with each producing at least 100 pea-sized stones. Of course, that was just a rough estimate. I never collected the gallstones in a colander or anything like that, though I read of people who did. I found the idea of collecting and individually counting gallstones simply nauseating. Anyway, supplementing with zinc and selenium was easy. I just started taking my set dosage amounts daily. The booster I needed to carefully monitor was the iodine. I was going to supplement with *nascent iodine* for thirty days. I chose nascent iodine because from the research it appeared that this form of iodine—its atomic form—is the most readily absorbed of all the iodine forms. Also, nascent iodine was widely used for a large number of health ailments before the advent of the huge pharmaceutical industry. Because of its impressive historical track record, and the fact that it is absorbed very quickly, I felt that nascent iodine was exactly the type of iodine I needed. I tried other forms of iodine later on, but I always came back to nascent iodine. It had a rather high price, but if my experiment worked, it would be worth every penny.

My plan was simple. I would supplement with iodine, gradually building up the amounts to 40-50 mg per day. After this, I would do an end-of-the-month liver flush and see what happens. What I was actually looking for, I wasn't exactly sure. I was hoping for a reduction in both the size and number of stones, but sometimes with scientific experimentation, you get results that are completely unexpected. Frankly, I didn't think thirty days of iodine supplementation was enough time to reboot a thyroid. From all I could find in the research, this would take six months to a year or more to accomplish. But this was a start in what I thought was the right direction.

As I started my iodine supplementation, slowly working my way up to the 40–50 mg ceiling, the first thing I noticed was that if I tried to increase my iodine dosage too quickly, I would get a Herxheimer reaction. This was actually a very encouraging sign. This told me that iodine was definitely doing something very good. Whether it was cleaning up mercury atoms from thyroid hormone receptor sites, rebooting a sluggish thyroid, or providing the raw materials for T4 and T3 construction, I did not know. But I did know from experience that a Herxheimer, although painful, was a sign that the detox protocol was probably working.

After thirty days of iodine supplementation, I had reached 40 grams of iodine per day. This was also the day of my fortieth flush, and I followed my standard routine. The night of the flush was uneventful, much like all of the others, but the next morning, I got my results. Here is my journal entry from that day: *Finished my fortieth flush today. Loads of small stones (like sand), but only a dozen or so stones about the size of a very small pea. Could be due to the effects of the iodine, but am unsure.*

I was extremely pleased with the results, but I tempered my enthusiasm with a reasonable amount of caution. Yes, I had gone from a pattern of a hundred or more pea-sized stones to only a dozen. This was encouraging, but I needed more evidence, just to be sure. I had to do it again. I had to keep taking the iodine and then do another liver flush in a month. In the meantime, I needed to do more research. I had some evidence now that I was on the right track, but I had many questions still unanswered. This was the first flush in years where I did not produce a large number of stones. If my thyroid reboot protocol was correct, the iodine supplementation had resulted in higher thyroxine amounts, which led to a more efficiently operating liver, particularly with regards to cholesterol metabolism. The increased thyroxine amounts also provided the key for the lock mechanism on the sphincter of Oddi.

If this was truly how it worked, I was curious to know why it worked. The only answer I could come up with was that I must have been seriously iodine deficient. This conclusion appeared to be highly improbable, and yet, my lack of stones on this fortieth flush seemed to indicate otherwise. If I was truly iodine deficient, how did I get that way? I felt that my diet was a healthy one, and I had faithfully taken high-quality multivitamin supplements, that included iodine in RDA amounts, for years. So, I was more than just a little confused at this seeming iodine deficiency. This was a big question that needed answering, and this is where I turned my attention to next.

# Chapter 34

# The Supplanting Agents

You may have noticed that the general tone of my writing has changed as you have progressed through this memoir. Considering that this memoir covers a twelve-year-period of my life, I suppose changes like these are natural. Maybe they should even be expected. The science I have been discussing has gradually become more sophisticated, because I had grown in my own understanding of the biochemical complexities involved in detoxification. But also, you may have noticed that this memoir has grown increasingly pessimistic in certain areas. This change accurately mirrors how I was thinking and feeling. To put it bluntly, I was becoming jaded.

Before I began my detoxing journey, I guess I had what you might call an inherent trust in the system. I believed that my food was healthy and nutritious, unless I specifically chose to eat junk food, which I frequently did. I also believed my air and water supply was, for the most part, clear and free of harmful contaminants and chemicals. When I did get sick, I believed that doctors, dentists, and even the government generally had my best interests in mind and would be there to take care of me. All of this was changing. It was not completely reversed, but I guess you could say it was now on a serious detour. As I advanced in my understanding of detoxification and started formulating my own various theories, I became increasingly skeptical concerning much of what modern medicine had to say about health, nutrition, and toxicity. And I had growing doubts that food manufacturers and their government regulatory counterparts had my best interests in mind. I know this sounds very negative, but I couldn't help it. After nearly ten years of struggling with toxicity, there were abundant aspects of the system that consistently disappointed me. This was particularly true as I began researching ways to clean up and detoxify a contaminated thyroid.

Very early in my research of the thyroid, I realized that adequate iodine was absolutely essential for proper thyroid functioning. Both the T3 and T4 thyroid hormone molecules require large amounts of iodine, and I needed plenty of these hormones to test and hopefully solve my gallstone problem. But as I studied, I quickly found that iodine deficiency is an enormous problem, worldwide. And it seemed highly likely that I was included in this group. I was seriously iodine deficient.

This was both an extremely surprising and exceedingly troubling revelation. How could something as vital to the human condition as iodine be lacking in a normal diet like mine? I knew iodine was important, and maybe that was the point. It was so important that I assumed other people were making sure that I was getting all of the iodine I needed. *Wasn't this the reason they put iodine in normal salt to begin with?* We take iodized salt because we recognize the importance of iodine in our diets. Well, I am fairly certain you see the flaw in my reasoning: *I assumed* other people were making sure that I was getting all of the iodine I needed. How many more times would I make this same mistake?

You would think that I would have caught on by now that the system was not constructed to take care of me. It was more of the other way around. I was steadily being prepared—or groomed if you will—to support and perpetuate the system.

What I found in the research on iodine deficiency simply shocked me. Do a web search on the World Health Organization's involvement in studying iodine deficiency. You too will be astounded. According to the WHO, approximately two billion people do not get a sufficient amount of iodine in their diets. *Two billion people—that's about a quarter of the world's population!* One study from the WHO states that large portions of the entire European continent are mildly iodine deficient. So if you were thinking that iodine deficiency is a third-world problem, think again. Iodine deficiency is

## THE SUPPLANTING AGENTS

a worldwide problem—that includes the United States and me and, in all probability, you too.

I began my research into iodine because I'd suspected a link between gallstones and thyroid function. Well, I'd found that link, but the whole notion of iodine deficiency being a worldwide problem was so much bigger than my little theories and experiments. It was a staggeringly large problem, and frankly, very difficult to process. But again, I needed to focus my attention to finish what I'd started. So I continued to research the notion of iodine deficiency and human toxicity.

I found that iodine plays a very prominent role in the human body's immune system. Iodine is even used by the body to ward off cancer. Yes, you read that correctly—*cancer*. I was shocked to find that iodine deficiency was strongly linked to cancer. Extremely curious at this connection, I dug deeper, and I found that iodine is involved in cancer prevention in an extremely interesting and powerful way.

Imagine you have a cell that, for one reason or another, has mutated. Its genetic code has been damaged, but not to the point of killing the cell. So the mutated cell continues to divide and multiply, despite its deformed or mutated state. Hordes of deformed or mutated cells swarming around will most likely be harmful to the body. But the body, in its brilliant design, has a self-destruct button for just such a situation. The technical term for this situation is "cellular apoptosis." Essentially what cellular apoptosis does is allow a mutated or deformed cell to kill itself. Once destroyed, obviously the cell can no longer multiply, and the body takes the raw materials of this exploded cell and recycles its atoms and molecules into something else. It's an amazingly efficient system that keeps the health and integrity of the body intact.

So what does this have to do with cancer? "Multiply in its mutated state" is a simple but accurate description of cancer. Now guess which element is required for cellular apoptosis to occur? *Iodine*. The element iodine is not only critical for life, it is also used to put mutated cells to death. No iodine; no cellular apoptosis. No cellular apoptosis means hordes of mutated cells are allowed to multiply. Of course, this does not mean that everyone who is iodine deficient will get cancer, but a definite link between iodine deficiency and cancer exists.

But there is more to the story. What I found extremely interesting is the actual locations of where the human body stores its surplus iodine amounts. Iodine is so important to overall life and health, the body actually keeps large iodine reserves. Iodine is stockpiled. The body's main concentration of iodine is, of course, the thyroid. But iodine is also found in large amounts in female breasts and in male prostates. Iodine. Apoptosis. Breasts. Prostate. Cancer. Death. It isn't hard to see the connection.

No iodine in storage would mean no cellular apoptosis. No apoptosis, and you could be dealing with cancer. And which cancers are absolutely devastating the world...particularly in industrialized nations? Exactly—prostate and breast cancer.

The effect of exploring the iodine-cancer relationship on me was profound. Iodine was no longer on the periphery for me. It stood at the center of my situation. If iodine was so critical in its interactions in warding off cancer, it had to have a powerful role in detoxing. My short thirty-day experiment showed that iodine supplementation was related to gallstones, but it also showed that I was, in all likelihood, seriously deficient in iodine.

I still needed an answer, or at least a theory, as to why so many people around the world were like me—iodine deficient. The most obvious answer was that the current dietary iodine intake was simply insufficient. A person requires X milligrams of iodine in their daily diet but consistently takes in an iodine amount that is less than X milligrams. After a period of time, they are iodine deficient. This makes sense in areas of the world where agricultural lands are worked so hard the trace minerals are depleted. It also makes sense that iodine deficiency might occur in areas where there is little knowledge or access to nutritional information and supplements. But I could not imagine that two billion people fit into one or both of these categories. It couldn't be that simple. It just didn't seem possible that one fourth of the world's population consistently gets less than a necessary minimum amount of iodine in their diets.

# THE SUPPLANTING AGENTS

Furthermore, I had been taking good multivitamins with mineral supplements for years, yet I still seemed to be seriously iodine deficient. For some unknown reason, I was also in this two-billion-person group. It couldn't have been all due to less than normal daily intake. No, I had a hunch it was a different mechanism—something much more subtle.

What if the problem was not getting too little iodine, but getting too much of something else that either prevents iodine from being absorbed by the body or accelerates its excretion from the body? *What could kick iodine out of the body or keep it from being absorbed?* I reasoned it had to be something extremely common; something found everywhere and presented to the public as good—or at least not harmful. If iodine deficiency was the globally huge problem that the WHO said it was, then it seemed reasonable that the cause of this deficiency must also be global. I was certain pollution in general was a causative factor—pollution always is. But I did not think that general pollution was the main factor. It had to be something ubiquitous and very specific in its targeting of iodine.

Well, after a significant amount of research on the subject and an intense examination of my own rather unique history with iodine-related chemicals, I developed a theory for much if not most of this iodine deficiency. But before I discuss this latest theory, it would be better to first to discuss how this theory actually came about.

I mentioned in a previous chapter that as I progressed in my detoxing, I grew increasingly sensitive to chemicals of various sorts. But I was not always like this. In fact, years earlier, I was fairly insensitive to some rather noxious chemicals. This included chlorine. I never really cared for the smell of chlorine, and as a chemistry teacher, I tried not to deal with this element in its gaseous form because it is an incredibly powerful and dangerous toxin. You may also recall, back in chapter one, I described the incident that for me was the beginning of my downward spiral of health. I was pulling some trash in a cart in my yard when my back suddenly went out. What I didn't mention in this chapter, because it wasn't relevant at the time, was that I collapsed next to the swimming pool we had in our backyard. Our home then had both an outdoor swimming pool and an indoor hot tub.

## DETOX MEMOIR

Back in those days, I was around chlorine all of the time. I had become so accustomed to the odor of chlorine that I hardly noticed it. I didn't think about it at the time, but I am fairly certain that getting used to the smell of a noxious poison like chlorine is not a good thing. In fact, this was probably a warning sign that something was wrong with my system. But back then, I was oblivious to it all.

Now, fast-forward several years to the time when I realized I had become so chemically sensitive. I was a sort of a human canary. My increasing sensitivity to chemical smells at that point stretched into the realm of super-sensitivity, and the smell of chlorine became more than just a slight nuisance. It had an irritating, almost choking effect on me. In just a few years I had gone from being completely oblivious to the smell of chlorine to being hypersensitive to it. Even the smell of chlorine in the municipal water supply was unmistakable. Tap water tasted absolutely terrible, and taking a hot shower was equally unpleasant because of the chlorine smell in the water vapor. This was a really strange time for me. I began to ask others about the smell of chlorine in their tap water, either for drinking or bathing. Nearly all of them said that they did not notice it at all or that it did not bother them. *How could the smell of a deadly poison like chlorine not bother you?* But to be fair, just a few years earlier, I was around chlorine all of the time, and it didn't bother me either.

What does all of this talk about chlorine have to do with my theory concerning iodine deficiency? Well, if you look at a periodic table, you will notice that iodine, the element that is absolutely essential for proper thyroid function, is in the same column as fluorine, chlorine, and bromine. These elements are called *halogens*. In their ionic (chemically active) forms, they called *halides*. I mentioned this earlier, but it's worth repeating: chemicals in the same column share many common chemical characteristics.

## THE SUPPLANTING AGENTS

Fluorine, chlorine, bromine, and iodine share many common chemical characteristics, not the least of which is that they are all poisonous. Yes, iodine (or iodide) is essential for all of the purposes I have already stated, but in large amounts, it can be lethal. Simply put, the elements in this column on the periodic table are very good at killing things.

Halides are very useful, but they can also be very deadly. This is one reason why chlorine, and oftentimes, fluoride are put in the municipal water supply—to kill bacteria and other pathogens. You undoubtedly know this. But what you might not know is that these three elements above iodine on the periodic table will also supplant iodine whenever and wherever they can. I don't want to get too technical here, but the key word is *electronegativity*. Here's an easy way to explain it. In a competition between a chlorine atom and an iodine atom, chlorine will win every time. Chlorine has a greater electronegativity. Fluorine is an even tougher competitor. It always wins in a competition. Fluorine has the highest electronegativity of any known element. So if we are ingesting fluorine, chlorine, and bromine, poor iodine will be supplanted and then excreted from the body.

It isn't natural for the body to relinquish an element as vital as iodine. Powerful chemical forces are needed for this to occur. Iodine is too important to the body for it to let iodine go without a struggle. But under the constant onslaught of fluorine and chlorine halides in the municipal water supply, and bromides in many types of breads and beverages, iodine amounts in the body slowly and steadily diminish. The body will receive the fluorine, chlorine, and bromine atoms because of their chemical similarity to iodine, but in the process, iodine becomes supplanted and is eventually removed from the body. Why does the body allow this? Because of electronegativity.

When I saw this big picture, it became very clear to me that any society that is as awash in halides as ours is will necessarily create

> *Any society that is as awash in halides as ours is will necessarily create an iodine deficiency within its populace.*

an iodine deficiency within its populace. It was simple chemistry being displayed on a very large stage. Hiding in plain sight and weakening my thyroid and shrinking my body's iodine stores were halides in air, food, and water, with ordinary tap water probably being the biggest offender. *Yes, ordinary tap water is a major cause of iodine deficiency.* How long would it take to create this iodine deficiency that would eventually lead to thyroid problems? I had no idea, but I knew it was only a matter of time. It was a slow kill of sorts—or as I call it, death by ten thousand pinpricks. Tap water is loaded with chlorine, so much so that you can actually smell it in many municipal water supplies. Many if not most municipalities also put fluoride in their water. This is double damage. If you think that you are safe because your municipal water supply is excellent, you might want to do some research on this. The fact is, most municipalities chlorinate and fluoridate their water. Some do so heavily, some lightly, but it's there all the same, and these halides will supplant iodine in the body without exception. If you are on well water or you have a whole-house system that filters out halides, you are much better off, but you're still not entirely free from iodine-supplanting agents. Why is this?

Think of all the foods and liquids you consume that contain water. Do you really believe that the food manufacturers that made your breakfast juice or that breakfast cereal or that can of soup that you had for lunch used *filtered water* to make their products? This is highly unlikely. Filtering huge volumes of water is a significant added expense that food companies typically try to avoid. Besides, the municipal water supply is supposed to be healthy and completely safe, so why should food manufacturers filter it anyway? To make matters worse, because these halides are placed in the municipal water supply, food manufacturers do not have to put halide amounts on their food labels. Have you ever seen fluoride or chlorine amounts on a food label? No, all you ever see is "water."

Furthermore, while there are trace amounts of other elements in the water, it is assumed that these are either beneficial (like magnesium, calcium, and iron), or if they are harmful (like arsenic, lead, and uranium), they are in such small amounts that their negative effects are presumed to be negligible. In either case, trace elements in the water never make it to a food label. Water is the world's greatest solvent, so having all sorts of elements dissolved in water is natural. But halides are different. The huge amount of halides in the municipal water supply are deliberately put there, and the result is anything but natural.

The main point of my iodine deficiency theory is simply this: people living in industrialized nations consume large amounts of halides daily. Each fluoride, chloride, and bromide ion that they take in potentially displaces vital iodine from the body. This is what happened to me. My iodine stores were diminished over time due to my frequent contact with chlorine from my swimming pool and hot tub and my lifelong ingestion of fluoride and chlorine in normal tap water. During those years when I had a very high exposure to chlorine due to frequent use and maintenance of the swimming pool and hot tub, my iodine depletion rate was significantly accelerated. Every day, I was being leached of iodine, until one day my thyroid weakened to a point where it could no longer produce thyroid hormones in the amounts that my body required. These halides, along with the daily influx of mercury leaching from my amalgam fillings, all worked synergistically to contaminate and incapacitate my thyroid—and I went down.

CHAPTER 35

# Predictability

One of the reasons I have always enjoyed science—and chemistry in particular—is because it is so predictable. People can lie. People can break the law. Chemicals can do neither of these things. Chemicals behave in very predictable and reproducible ways. Because they do, I was thoroughly convinced the fluorine and chlorine I had been eating, drinking, bathing in, and brushing with my entire life weakened my thyroid. It seemed pretty clear that if my thyroid was perfectly healthy, then these chemicals were breaking the law. But chemicals can't do that. Powerful halides supplant weaker ones, and that means fluorine and chlorine replace iodine. End of story.

This was a terribly inconvenient truth, because it put into question or directly contradicted many things that I had thought were true for a very long time. But once I really got hold of this idea, I just could not see any other way of explaining some of my conditions. If you are skeptical of these conclusions, and you should be, I suggest you do some research on your own. If you start with a web search header like "chlorine and thyroid problems" or "fluoride and thyroid problems" and do some research yourself, you may see things quite differently.

> If you are skeptical of these conclusions, and you should be, I suggest you do some research on your own... you may see things quite differently.

For my part, I was convinced I was on the right track. I had seen a vast improvement with my gallstone issue due to my thyroid boosters. My fortieth liver flush produced very few large stones at all. After several months, I did my forty-first and forty-second flushes with the same results. Very few stones. This was an incredible improvement from previous flushes, where the number of stones was in the hundreds. Then I decided to flip the experiment. Over the course of several more months, I would not take my thyroid boosters and see what the result was. The only iodine that I received during those months was through my regular diet, and the small microgram amounts that were included in my multivitamin. After this time of testing was over, I was ready for flush forty-three. The results were hundreds of stones! The stones returned when I did not take my thyroid boosters, which were 40 mg of zinc, 200 mcg of selenium, and 40–50 mg of iodine.

This small experiment was all the convincing that I needed. A strong connection existed between gallstones and the thyroid, and the gallstone problem could be remedied with thyroid boosting supplements. This discovery gave my confidence an incredible and much-needed lift. And it also gave me the confidence I needed to proceed with boosting my children's thyroid functioning. As with me, my children's multivitamins provided all of the necessary nutrients, especially the selenium and zinc, to boost the thyroid. But the main booster, iodine, was sorely lacking in their multivitamin. So, just as I had done for myself, I added an iodine supplement to their diet, but only at a fraction of the dosage that I was taking. I also began tapering off the normal chelating supplements they had been taking for years. I was fairly confident at this point that most of the toxic metals were greatly reduced, except in the most stubborn areas like the thyroid hormone receptor sites, and I was curious to see the effects that the thyroid boosters would have on their next lab report. If my theory was correct, the boosters would help clean up and clear away the mercury that was currently disrupting normal thyroid function. This would result in a strengthened thyroid, which would then actively work with the other systems to more effectively detox the entire body.

A stronger and cleaner thyroid also meant a higher metabolic rate, which is extremely important to young, growing bodies. My kids were growing and gaining weight, and I wanted them to gain this weight in the right way and in the right places. As an added bonus, the extra iodine would also push out of their bodies some of those awful halides they had been taking in their entire lives.

| POTENTIALLY TOXIC ELEMENTS (8 Year Old ♀) | | | | |
|---|---|---|---|---|
| | RESULT µg/g | RANGE | PERCENTILE 68th | 95th |
| Aluminum | 11 | <12.0 | | |
| Antimony | <0.01 | <0.080 | | |
| Arsenic | 0.045 | <0.120 | | |
| Bismuth | 0.013 | <2.0 | | |
| Cadmium | 0.016 | <0.150 | | |
| Lead | 0.10 | <2.0 | | |
| Mercury | <0.03 | <1.10 | | |
| Uranium | 0.14 | <0.060 | | |
| Nickel | 0.18 | <0.40 | | |
| Silver | 0.02 | <0.10 | | |
| Tin | 0.07 | <0.30 | | |
| Titanium | 0.31 | <1.00 | | |
| Total Toxic Representation | | | | |

After about a year of taking the boosters, I sent new hair samples to the lab. I was mainly interested in my daughter's data. As I stated earlier, my daughter was the far more toxic of my two children because she was younger, and therefore carried a heavier toxic burden. When I received the results back from the lab, I simply could not stop smiling. I was blown away with the improvement I saw in this report, particularly when it was compared to what we had received from the lab only a year earlier. Although I could not prove it, the evidence seemed to strongly indicate that the thyroid boosters had worked wonderfully well for my children.

It had been nearly four years since I began these basic detox protocols with my children, and I was certain that they were happier and healthier than ever before. Obviously there was still room for improvement, but when I considered what these lines may have looked like had I done nothing for them these past four years, there was no comparison. The data from this hair analysis was excellent, and it further solidified my thinking concerning the thyroid and its critical role in detoxing the entire body. I was also greatly encouraged by the speed of it all. My daughter had only been taking the thyroid boosters for about a year, and her improvement during this fourth year was simply astonishing.

To summarize, my daughter took mostly mild, over-the-counter, chelating supplements. During the fourth year, she took very few of the chelators, focusing on the daily multivitamin and iodine supplements to boost her thyroid performance. Even if I was wrong with most of my theories in this memoir, obviously something was now going very right.

| Toxin | Original Level | After 46 Months | % Increase or Decrease |
|---|---|---|---|
| Aluminum | 38.0 | 11.0 | 71% Decrease |
| Antimony | 0.17 | <0.01 | 99% Decrease |
| Arsenic | 0.043 | 0.045 | 5% Increase |
| Bismuth | 0.84 | 0.013 | 98% Decrease |
| Cadmium | 0.21 | 0.016 | 92% Decrease |
| Lead | 1.30 | 0.10 | 92% Decrease |
| Mercury | 0.14 | <0.003 | 99% Decrease |
| Uranium | 0.098 | 0.14 | 43% Increase |
| Nickel | 1.10 | 0.18 | 84% Decrease |
| Silver | 17.0 | 0.02 | 99% Decrease |
| Tin | 0.61 | 0.03 | 95% Decrease |
| Titanium | 5.0 | 0.31 | 94% Decrease |

As I reflected further on this data, I was grateful that I had started detoxing my kids very early on in life. I was now about ten years into my researching and experimentation. But what good would all of my research have been if I was the only one to benefit from it? If I completely regained my own health, but my kids were dreadfully sick due to toxicity—what was the point? One person put it this way: "The benefits of science are not for the scientist, but for humanity." I am not calling myself a scientist. I'm not sure I qualify for that title. As I have already indicated, my doctoral degree is in education. As an educator, I enjoy helping people. I had helped myself. And now I was helping my kids detoxify their bodies. This gave me immense satisfaction. I didn't look at the figures on the hair analysis form as mere abstract numbers. Those numbers represented a better future.

Like any parent, I wanted a bright future for my children. I did not want them or anyone else to be bound and afflicted with the same types of horrible health issues that I had to contend with. And from all that I could see now, they wouldn't be.

# Chapter 36

# Not a Chance

One of the things that really bothers me is that most people seem almost resigned to the fact that sickness will come to them on a regular basis. It is almost as if sickness were just a matter of chance, mixed in with a bit of genetics, and sautéed with a dash of lifestyle choices. Of course genetics and lifestyle choices play critical roles in one's health and sickness, but I don't see how chance comes into the equation at all. I see chance as simply a word we use when we don't know what the causal factor is.

I looked at my own condition with this same type of reasoning, particularly after I was making great strides with my thyroid boosters. *Besides the thyroid, what else would logically be damaged by a daily barrage of halide ingestion?* It seemed only reasonable to conclude that decades of drinking and bathing in water that was conditioned with fluoride and chlorine must have had a negative impact on my digestive system. And working with and around chlorine during those years that I had a hot tub and swimming pool at my home didn't help my health either.

We use chlorine to clean our sinks and tubs—and though this is a highly diluted solution of chlorine, it does the job quite effectively. Chlorine kills mold, fungus, and bacteria almost instantly. As I mentioned before, halides are very good at killing things. That is the point. Whatever chlorine does for my hot tub, it will also do to my intestines, because chemicals obey the law, 100 percent of the time. There was no *chance* about it. Chlorine kills. So what were the long-term effects of daily drinking a few liters of fluoridated and chlorinated water on normal intestinal flora? I started to wonder.

Most of the bacteria in the intestines are extremely useful, even essential. Yet I had been ingesting daily, for decades, chemicals that are harmful to this friendly bacteria. Because of my chronic battle with gallstones, I suspected that my intestinal pH was a mess due to the lack of adequate bile flow. Instead of 500 ml of bile flowing through the intestines on a daily basis, I had an unknown lesser amount flowing because of the blockage caused by the stones. This, in conjunction with problems with the sphincter of Oddi, caused a veritable "bile drought" in the intestines. I knew this was not good for intestinal flora, and it probably contributed to my chemical sensitivities, food allergies, nutrient deficiencies, and overall malaise.

I had not looked into the question of healthy intestinal flora too much earlier because, frankly, my attention was primarily on other aspects of my deteriorating health. But now that the liver and thyroid problems had vastly improved, the issue of healthy intestinal flora was right in front of me, and I couldn't ignore it any longer. I was certain I was loaded with harmful halides, and it was now time to detox myself of all of the chlorine, fluorine, and bromine in my system.

However, just as I was starting to prepare for another round of detoxing, things suddenly got much easier. As I did the research on halide detox protocols, I found that the answer to this problem was something I was already doing—iodine supplementation. Yes, iodine is supplanted by these three chemicals, but in sufficiently high enough doses, the opposite will also occur. Fifty mg of iodine daily was a high enough dose to push the excess fluorides, chlorides, and bromides out of my system. Of course, I was also taking my other thyroid boosters, zinc and selenium, in order to keep my thyroid hormone levels in balance, because 50 mg of iodine is a high daily intake. From all I could find in the research, doing this for six months to a year would do wonders for reversing much of the damage done due to decades of ingesting fluorides (water, toothpaste), chlorides (water), and bromides (bread and other foods). After a year or so of this high iodine supplementary amount, I would drop the dosage down to a daily maintenance dosage of around 8 mg per day.

At this point, you may be thinking what I have thought many times as I was going through my reasoning and research on detoxification. *There is no way to live on planet earth without being regularly exposed to harmful chemicals.* Toxins are all around us. Even with all of the safeguards I was putting in place, I knew there were many things beyond my control in terms of the toxins in the air, water, and soil. But there were also many things that I could control, that I simply did not want to.

For example, there were foods that I just didn't want to give up. How could I control how much potassium bromate was in that hot dog or hamburger bun I ate—if it was in the bun at all? What about the halides in that pizza I was eating? I could not control what the food manufacturers did, but I certainly could control what I put in my mouth. I did not want to live in some self-constructed bubble, free from all toxins in the environment. That's not living—it is existing, but only just barely.

If I wanted to live even a semi-normal existence, I had to resign myself to the fact that breathing in and eating some toxins were a part of everyday life. That is just the world we have now. This is why putting safeguards in place, like iodine supplementation, which could operate in the background, was so vitally important. I wasn't about to stop swimming in a chlorinated pool from time to time just because I would be swimming in a toxic chemical. Nor was I going to stop eating out at my favorite pizza place because I had a strong suspicion that the flour they used to make the pizza dough contained potassium bromate. I was satisfied that if I kept my iodine armor on with regular low-dosage maintenance levels, along with the selenium and zinc, it would suffice to not only protect me from thyroid damage, it would also work to continually strengthen my thyroid and immune system.

My research into iodine also had some other benefits that were actually quite surprising. I am not a good cook. But since most restaurants had been off-limits to me for several years now, I was slowly improving in this area by reason of necessity. One of the things I found as I developed my cooking skills was how good sea salt and deep-mined salt tastes. I grew up on iodized salt and was very accustomed to its taste. But when I compared the taste of iodized salt to that of unrefined sea salt or deep-mined salt, I found out what *real* salt tastes like. Iodized salt has a harsh, almost bitter taste in comparison to these other types of salts. But there is more. If you remember, during my research, I started to question the notion that much of the iodine I really needed would be provided by iodized salt. Now I was convinced that it was absolutely impossible to get sufficient iodine amounts by simply garnishing one's food with iodized salt. Iodized salt may keep goiter away, but as far as I could see, those iodine amounts were just barely above the starvation threshold for any thyroid. Furthermore, I was convinced that meeting much of the body's iodine requirements by way of iodized salt would give anyone far more sodium in their diet than what could ever be considered healthy.

Iodized salt is a combination of sodium, chlorine, and iodine. As has already been noted, iodine and chlorine are in the same chemical family. Though they share similar chemical characteristics, being bonded to one another is not natural for these two elements. Iodizing normal salt has to be done artificially. But being synthetically generated is a bad starting point for any kind of food. Forcing the iodine atom to bond with a sodium chloride molecule requires raising the temperature of the chemical mixture to over 1,000° Fahrenheit. That sounds "all natural," doesn't it? I suspected I had found yet another snake-oil trap, with iodized salt being the bait, and I was not disappointed.

> But being synthetically generated is a bad starting point for any kind of food.

The term "bioavailability" means exactly what it says: it is a measure of how much of a substance will be available to support life. I suspected that the bioavailability of a nutrient like iodine would be very low in iodized salt, and from all I could find in the research, it was about 10 percent or less. This is fairly typical of all synthetic food. It was very high on hype and extremely low on health.

As I said before, one thing that I had learned over and over again in my detox journey is that anytime man tries to "create" food, it ends of having some sort of toxic side effect. I have never seen an exception to this. God created food, and He put it in nature. It was good. Humans come along and try to improve on it. This is bad. For example, humans take sugar and say "Sugar? Don't you know how bad sugar is for you? Our scientists have developed something better, and we call it *Sweet X*. You need to eat Sweet X instead of sugar."

Have you heard this reasoning before? It is an extremely common sales technique, but it is not an honest one. And of course, we all know how the story ends. It might take years, even decades, but eventually we hear stories about how Sweet X actually causes high blood pressure, liver and kidney failure, cancer, brain hemorrhaging, and so on. Artificial sweeteners, artificial colors, artificial flavors, even the ubiquitous "natural flavors" are all in the same category. They all have nasty side effects. This means that they must contain toxic components that the liver must make specific molecules and enzymes for in order to break the toxic components down so that they don't poison you. This doesn't sound like food to me. It sounds more like another chemical time bomb. Sooner or later, this bomb will explode, and then we will all look around at each other and wonder what went wrong.

CHAPTER 37

# Different Problem, Same Solution

In some ways, doing research is like exploring an iceberg. On the surface, an issue may look relatively small—even harmless. But the more you look, the more things reveal themselves, and you begin to see the actual magnitude of the issue. What began as something small is suddenly monumental. This is the way it was for me and fluoride. I was making great strides in reducing my exposure to chemicals that would deplete the vital iodine in my body. I knew that fluorine, chlorine, and bromine were to be avoided, and I had put several safeguards in place to reduce my exposure. I had installed a whole-house water filtration system that filtered all of the chlorine and much of the fluoride out of our tap water. I brushed with non-fluoridated toothpaste or just plain baking soda with a small amount of peppermint oil for its antibacterial qualities, and for its fresh minty taste.

This was all good, but when friends and family members asked about fluorine or its ionic form, fluoride, I had trouble answering their questions. Of course, most of my research was with chlorine, not fluorine. Chlorine was the main halogen I was focused on because I was around it so much, especially during those years of living in the house with the swimming pool and hot tub. Also, chlorine's powerful taste and odor had really annoyed me when I was in my human canary days of super sensitivity. But fluoride in the municipal water supply has neither taste nor odor, so it had really been under my radar. The only reason it got my attention was because it was in the same family as chlorine, bromine, and iodine, and I knew that chemical families share common chemical characteristics. But what did I really know about fluorine and its ionic form, fluoride? Honestly, not that much.

I recall getting doses of fluoride at my dentist's office when I was a child. I also received doses of fluoride when I was in elementary school. Our school was so concerned for our dental health that they even brought in dental professionals to administer fluoride treatments to us during the school day. I remember being given a choice of either grape or cherry flavored fluoride. It had a strange, sour taste, but it wasn't too bad. I was told this was good for my teeth and would get rid of things that would lead to cavities. A cavity, of course, was every child's nightmare, because it necessitated a trip to the dreaded dentist. Most local governments in the United States put fluoride in their municipal water supplies for the same reason. The same was true with brushing your teeth with fluoride. *Take your fluoride every day or face the dentist's drill tomorrow.*

> Take your fluoride every day or face the dentist's drill tomorrow.

Looking back now, this all seemed like extremely cleverly packaged propaganda, based on fear and ignorance, not science. And this package was sold to a naïve general public. Just think about this question for a moment. Is putting the most powerful and dangerous halide in existence into a young person's mouth really necessary to prevent tooth decay? As I began to delve into the research on fluoride supplementation, I started to have some serious questions concerning the efficacy of it all. I began to have that sadly familiar and foreboding feeling that this was déjà vu all over again.

Fluoride is a deadly toxin. As a chemistry teacher, this is one element that I deliberately never worked with. It was just too dangerous. I had in my science lab a highly concentrated form of hydrochloric acid. I almost never used this acid in its highly concentrated form, and always took extreme caution when I diluted it. One slip or spill of that stuff and I or my students could be in serious trouble. This was hydrochloric acid. *Hydrofluoric* acid is even more dangerous. Hydrofluoric acid is so powerful it can even dissolve glass. Clearly, fluoride is a chemical that is not to be messed with. Yet I had trusted that the dental experts knew what they were doing.

But as you know by now, I had been burned by this trust many times before. Now, fluoride was at the center of my attention, and I began to research its use. To my great surprise, I found that fluoride and mercury have a significant number of commonalities with each other—all of which are bad. Consider the list I compiled:

1. Both mercury (Hg) and fluorine (F) toxicities are difficult to diagnose, and therefore have slipped by mainstream medicine's notice for decades.
2. Both of these powerful toxins are given to the public in large amounts. Mercury is given to the public in foods, vaccines, and dental fillings. Fluorine is given to the public in the municipal water supply, toothpaste, and in dental offices.
3. Both chemicals are proven amplifiers for other toxins. Both mercury and fluorine have a remarkable and disastrous ability to amplify the effects of other toxins in the body. Whatever is wrong with the human system will be made exponentially worse with the addition of either mercury or fluorine.
4. Both of these toxins are incredibly powerful chemical disrupters. Fluorine has no equal in terms of its electronegative capacity, and mercury has a powerful affinity for sulfur and selenium. It naturally bonds to and disrupts the normal function of proteins.
5. Both fluorine and mercury can pass the critical brain-blood barrier, which is an unusual quality for a chemical. This means fluorine and mercury can cause a range of neurological issues—from mild brain fog to insanity.
6. Mercury shuts down the toxic excretion system via the liver, and fluorine does much the same with the thyroid. The thyroid is also attacked by mercury, as mercury atoms can bind to thyroid hormone

receptor sites, disrupting thyroid function in yet another powerful and destructive way.
7. Both mercury and fluorine have the iniquitous history of being used to deliberately and slowly poison people. Tales of mercury being used to poison people abound throughout history. Fluorine is more of a newcomer in the poisoning department because it is much more difficult to synthesize and purify. But it has the infamous reputation of being used by the Nazis during World War II. Nazi prison camp administrators put fluoride into the prisoners' water supply to keep the prison population docile.

*Keep the prisoners docile with fluoride? That's a good one. Use a colorless, odorless, and flavorless powerful toxin that can melt away a prisoner's willpower to resist and escape, and put it into their water supply.* Genius. Pure evil, but genius nonetheless. Again, if you doubt or question any of these claims, you know what you need to do: research it yourself. Despite what the Nazis did or did not do with their prisoners, the truth is powerful halides supplant weaker ones. This is a chemical law.

Though this law was used against me, I had now turned it to my advantage. And here is the beauty of this whole fluoride-mercury connection. If mercury and fluoride were truly amplifiers of other toxins in the body, which I believed was true, then it seemed logical that the reduction of fluoride and mercury would lead to an exponential decrease in the other toxin levels in the body. Clean up the liver and the thyroid, and good things will happen very quickly. This is what was currently happening to me, and now I understood more fully why it was happening.

CHAPTER 38

# Dipping Seven Times in the Jordan

I started my journey with four goals in mind. I wanted to find a detox protocol that was easy to understand, easy to do, inexpensive, and quick in its operation. At this point, I had in place the first three elements, but not the fourth. I had been struggling with finding answers to my health problems for ten years now, so obviously I had not found something that was "fairly quick in its operation."

One thing that I knew would speed the detoxification process was what I referred to as "constructive redundancies." These were aspects of my detox protocol that served multiple purposes. For example, while iodine supplementation worked to reboot a polluted thyroid, it was also a potent mercury chelator. Iodine also provided a powerful boost to metabolism and to the immune system. It was also critical for supplanting harmful halides and halogens like fluoride, chlorine, and bromine. So my iodine supplementation was an extremely useful constructive redundancy.

Reestablishing normal bile flow was another such constructive redundancy. Restoring bile flow meant eliminating or at least alleviating a serious amount of liver congestion, which I knew would provide enormous health benefits. Moreover, reestablishing normal bile flow would again give the body the ability to properly digest fats, metabolize cholesterol, and enhance the movement of waste through the intestines. Furthermore, restoring normal bile flow was essential for creating an intestinal environment that was perfectly pH-balanced for the growth of good bacteria. I loved these constructive redundancies because they were so efficient and could save untold amounts of time, money, and energy. Plus, these redundancies fit in nicely with the Occam's razor philosophical paradigm. Actually, things were moving along quite nicely now. I was making gains in my health, my understanding of detoxification, and in my perspective. I summarized some of these gains in a chart, which is shown here.

| PROBLEM | SOLUTION | STATUS |
|---|---|---|
| Decrease the inflow of new mercury and halide ions into my system. | Complete dental revision; dietary adjustments; whole-house water filtration system installed. | Done |
| Mobilize mercury from body tissues and have it excreted. | Numerous liver flushes to restore normal bile flow, putting glutathione again into circulation; use of chelation supplements; iodine supplementation; increase raw food consumption. | Done |
| Recurring Herxheimer reactions | 1-2 heaping teaspoons of activated charcoal dissolved in black cherry juice. | On an as-needed basis |
| Liver returning to a congested state | Standard liver flush; iodine supplementation to provide for thyroxine production. | 1–2 flushes per year |
| Clean up thyroid of mercury so that the amounts of T3 and T4 are produced in their proper proportions. | Multivitamins with nascent iodine supplementation, working slowly up to 40–50 mg per day with selenium (200 mcg) and zinc (40 mg) daily for at least six months. | Done |

| PROBLEM | SOLUTION | STATUS |
|---|---|---|
| Bring iodine levels to maintenance dosage, to neutralize environmental halide exposure and to avoid hyper- or hypothyroid conditions. | Multivitamin, which includes trace elements. Iodine maintenance dose of 4–8 mg per day, periodically add additional selenium and zinc supplements. | Doing |
| Intestinal dysbiosis (flora levels are highly unbalanced). Intestinal pH is probably unbalanced, causing good bacterial death and bad bacterial, fungal, and intestinal parasite growth. | As bile flow rates are restored to their normal levels, pH should be restored to normal levels, which should cause the intestinal flora balance to be reestablished; supplement with a potent probiotic. | Doing, but definitely am missing something here. |

This chart was helpful in keeping me focused, and it assisted me in seeing what I needed to do next. I knew which of the protocols I had done actually worked, both because of the numbers I received from my lab data and by how I was feeling. And of course, I knew what had not worked, and I didn't waste any more time or money on those things. In short, I felt that I was getting close to the endpoint…but I wasn't there yet.

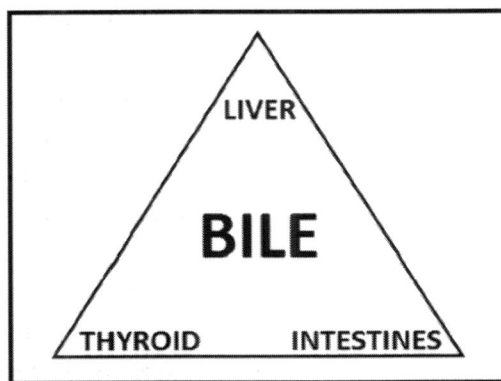

I had come a very long way, from being basically clueless concerning toxicity to making solid gains in my health. Over the years I also formulated several theories as to why my health had crashed, and how I could recover from that crash. One of the most important theories that I created was what I called the liver toxicity cycle, or LTC. While I still felt the LTC was accurate, I now knew it was incomplete. For example, the LTC was not able to explain the actual cause of gallstones. When I learned that the primary cause for gallstones was a thyroid hormone issue, I knew I had to revise my LTC. After assessing my own situation, along with a considerable amount of additional research, I clearly saw that the intestines also played an integral role in detoxing. With these ideas in mind, I expanded the LTC theory into an elegantly simple detoxification meta-theory, which I call the "detox triangle."

At the center of the detox triangle was bile. I put bile at the center because I saw it as the single most important aspect of detoxing. Who would have thought that lowly bile would hold such a prominent role in the body's overall health? Certainly not me. Well, not until I spent nearly a decade looking for the elusive answers to this detox puzzle. Now I saw things completely differently. Common bile was anything but common— it was absolutely critical for detoxing to occur because the bile carries glutathione, the body's master molecule for detoxification. Glutathione-rich bile travels through the liver, gallbladder, past the pancreas, and into the intestines, detoxing everything along its path. When bile is flowing in normal volumes, upward of a half-liter per day, the liver is able to detox itself, the intestines, and everything in between, while at the same time keeping the vital intestinal pH in its normal range. Everything is in perfect stasis with normal bile flow.

However, when bile is backed up due to gallstones, which I believed was due to toxicity and abnormal thyroid operation, this perfect stasis is destroyed. Once the stasis is gone, health problems due to toxicity begin to manifest themselves. But the all-important question was, how can someone know for certain if they have an adequate bile flow?

I could find no other way but a liver flush. I really dug into the research on this question, but the answer remained the same. There is currently no known way to measure bile flow without extensive surgery. Because there is no currently known diagnostic tool available to measure bile flow, bile's importance in digestion and detoxification is exceedingly underestimated and misunderstood in mainstream medical circles. This misunderstanding has made the cholecystectomy (gallbladder removal) one of the world's most common surgeries. When you consider the actual mechanics of gallstone obstruction, it is clear that the cholecystectomy is a clumsy workaround at best. A cholecystectomy actually ignores the real problem and treats only a portion of the symptoms. Gallstones don't even originate in the gallbladder—they originate in the liver. So why remove an entire organ that is downstream from the actual problem?

The point is, this extreme difficulty in being able to directly measure bile flow has indirectly caused bile to move to the periphery of mainstream medicine's detox equation; whereas I believe it belongs front and center. Bile is the key in the detox triangle because if bile production goes down, a person's toxicity goes up. It's that simple.

> Bile is the key in the detox triangle because if bile production goes down, a person's toxicity goes up. It's that simple.

At the top of the detox triangle is the body's chemical factory—the liver. The liver is both a chemical factory and the body's main toxic chemical filter. The liver is preeminent in terms of keeping the body as toxin-free as possible, and that is why I put the liver at the top of the triangle. Approximately two liters of blood pass through the liver every minute for filtering. Obviously, cleaning this organ at the beginning of any detox journey was a logical first step. Doing all of those liver flushes and adding chelation supplements to my diet had accomplished this liver cleaning, and I had outstanding results in my blood work and hair analyses as evidence of this.

The second tip of the detox triangle is another filter, the thyroid. People don't normally look at the thyroid this way but I did. I see the thyroid as a powerful filter, because the entire human blood supply passes through the thyroid once every hour. If toxins like mercury are circulating in the blood, many of these toxins are filtered out and deposited on thyroid tissues. This is especially true with the selenium-rich tissue making up the thyroid hormone receptor sites. Because mercury has a powerful attraction to selenium, mercury flowing in the blood will eventually be deposited on delicate thyroid tissues. I took thyroid rebooting supplements for the purposes of cleaning and revitalizing my thyroid, and then tested my theory that gallstones are directly related to the thyroid hormone thyroxine. This first reboot worked, as I produced almost no stones with my next liver flush. I repeated my reboot protocol two more times with two subsequent liver flushes and the results were the same—almost no stones. Then I stopped taking my thyroid boosters for several months to again test the thyroid reboot theory. My next liver flush produced perhaps a hundred stones, some of which were pea-sized or larger! This was all the confirmation that I needed for my little theory. I resumed a maintenance-level dosage of thyroid boosters for a healthy thyroid, and of course to keep the gallstones away. I continue to do so to this present day.

Like the other two tips of the detox triangle, the third tip is also a filter, though like the thyroid, perhaps not in the traditional sense. The intestines filter our foods, with the good nutrients being absorbed into the blood and the waste material being excreted. This part of my triangle was, at this point in my journey, the least understood and least researched. I had hoped that once normal bile flow was reestablished, the glutathione-rich bile would be sufficient enough to thoroughly detoxify the intestines. I was also supplementing with high-grade probiotics, which I hoped would successfully colonize within the intestines, and thereby reestablish normal intestinal flora levels.

I knew very well that harmful intestinal flora, bacteria, and parasites produce horrible toxins like ammonia, ethanol, carbon monoxide, and acetaldehyde. I was hoping that my rebooted thyroid and clean liver would eliminate the need for any additional detox strategy to be applied to the intestines. Now I was beginning to suspect that I was very wrong about this. I still had a few lingering symptoms that stubbornly held onto me. As

I had not given much attention to the intestines before, I realized I needed to do so now. So, I dove back into the research looking for the remaining elusive answers.

This had been a long journey—much longer than what I had ever anticipated. I had spent ten years of my life looking for solutions. During the first five years, I'd found very little worth holding onto, except of course, what *not* to do. However, the following five years were extremely productive and brought about many changes, most of which were incredibly positive. This was important, because all of this detoxing and experimentation was a lonely business at times. Having made so many wrong decisions in the past, it was extremely encouraging to finally see data indicating that I was on the right track.

My energy levels—including strength and stamina—were now excellent. My immune system was vastly improved, and I required much less sleep than what I used to need. I also required less food. This was a very surprising but extremely welcome benefit. I frequently ate just two meals a day, and sometimes only one. I drank plenty of high-quality water throughout the day, and I never snacked. My body felt fit and trim, and my mind was clear. All of that horrible brain fog and depression, which seemed at times to come and go with a will of its own, was now long gone. Mentally, I felt as sharp as I had ever been, and my ability to recall facts and compute data was excellent. Furthermore, I almost never had an outbreak in hives, and I hadn't had an incident of swelling in a very long time.

To sum things up, I had experienced over the last few years what can only be described as a major body upgrade. I was feeling tremendous nearly all of the time. But I was still not completely clear of symptoms.

As shown in this chart, I was still sensitive to monosodium glutamate (MSG). I knew this because I would occasionally test my sensitivity by deliberately eating foods that contained MSG. Unfortunately, I failed my own personal MSG test every time. Each time I ate food with MSG, within six hours or so, I would experience an allergic reaction in the form of hives or swelling. The good news was that I did not seem to react nearly as violently to MSG as I had in the past. This was good, but it was painfully clear that I was still sensitive to this horrible chemical food additive. Still, seeing that MSG was not healthy to consume anyway, this was not a huge problem. This did limit my menu choices at any given restaurant, but by now my willpower was far greater than my desire to just eat anything that looked good on a menu.

| SYMPTOM | IMPROVEMENT |
|---|---|
| MSG sensitivity | Moderate |
| Sinusitis | Excellent |
| Immune system | Excellent |
| Nausea | Moderate |
| Lower-back pain | Excellent |
| Arthritic foot pain | Excellent |
| Brain Fog | Excellent |
| Hives, rash, swelling | Very Good |
| Numbness in toes | Very Good |
| Chronic fatigue | Excellent |
| Chemical sensitivity | Very Good |
| Testosterone levels | Excellent |

Another symptom I still had was a red, bumpy, itchy rash in both underarm areas. I initially thought this rash was a reaction to the deodorant I was using. But after changing the brand several different times and seeing no improvement, I just ignored the problem. The rash was annoying however, and it got worse if I scratched it. To be completely candid, however, in comparison to all of my other symptoms, the underarm rash never ranked very high on my priority list. But now that most of my other symptoms had gone away, it now had my attention.

But probably the most annoying symptom that I was still dealing with was some occasional nausea after eating a meal. It wasn't a regular occurrence, but it was rather strange. I called it my "sour stomach," because that is what it felt like. I did not believe it had anything to do with the food I ate, because both healthy and not-so-healthy food could give me a sour stomach from time to time. With this symptom, and a few other minor ones still present, I knew I had missed something significant along the way. And I had a feeling these last few symptoms had to do with the intestines because this was the one major area of detoxification that I had not yet directly addressed.

The intestines are a type of filter too, just like the liver and thyroid, and I wanted to clean out all of my filters. I thought that the intestines would improve as my bile flow improved. I felt that supplementing with a good probiotic would also help recolonize intestinal flora to their normal levels. After more research, I became convinced that this approach to cleaning up the intestines was far too passive. I also found in the research some rather interesting information concerning my underarm rash. This rash could quite possibly be evidence of a fungus. Fungi love dark, warm, and moist environments. This perfectly described the underarm area. It also perfectly described the intestinal environment. This, along with my continued MSG sensitivity, told me that all was not completely well with my intestines. These seemed like fairly good clues that I probably had an unhealthy amount of intestinal hitchhikers who were living off the fat of the land—or in this case, the fat of the man. What I'm referring to here is a fungal overgrowth, which is a type of intestinal parasite.

*Human parasites.* Just the thought of this was revolting. And yet, after doing a significant amount of research, internal parasites seemed like a very real and very horrible possibility. An intestinal system that was out of its normal pH range for a long period of time would be an extremely attractive place for parasites to entrench themselves. Furthermore, parasites are living organisms. They are not like toxic metals. Once the mercury, aluminum, arsenic, nickel, or whatever toxic element you can think of is removed, it is gone for good. Because internal parasites are alive, they have the unique ability to continually contaminate the human system with daily doses of their insidious toxic waste products.

Parasites have the incredible ability to create a perpetual cycle of toxicity that theoretically could last a lifetime. The more I looked into this disgusting hypothesis, the more convinced I became that parasites were in fact the final missing piece to my detox puzzle. How did I become so convinced of this? Like any detective who gets a bit lost and confused in the virtual forest of data, I simply retraced my steps and went back to the beginning.

My troubles began with what I believe to be the most powerfully toxic element on the planet: mercury. I was born with mercury in my organs from my mother and probably my maternal grandmother. I also had all my vaccinations as a child, most of which contained thimerosal, a chemical additive that is almost 50 percent mercury by weight. And of course, I'd had mercury amalgam fillings placed in my mouth at a very young age. Mercury, whether from prenatal exposure, vaccinations, foods, or leaching from amalgam fillings, destroys or damages everything in its path. This includes the parietal cells of the stomach.

Parietal cells are the specialized cells of the stomach that make hydrochloric acid, which normally would be strong enough to kill any parasites (or parasite eggs) found in food. It seemed reasonable to assume that after more than twenty years of swallowing mercury-laced saliva, my parietal cells were probably not in the best of shape. That would, in turn, weaken the quality and quantity of hydrochloric acid needed for digestion and for the destruction of any parasites and their eggs that might be in my food. With parasites and their eggs now able to survive the stomach acid, they could enter the bloodstream, the intestines, and go anywhere in the body.

Parasites that entered the intestine would have to face the human body's second line of defense, the bile. Because normal bile is highly alkaline, or caustic, most or all of the remaining parasites and their eggs should have been destroyed. But I had learned long ago that a toxic person's bile flow is greatly diminished due to gallstones that were brought on by the toxicity itself. So bile as a second line of defense, like the stomach's hydrochloric acid, was in all likelihood, greatly compromised. The final line of defense against a parasitic attack, attachment, and entrenchment was the body's immune system.

But I had known for some time that mercury has a powerful ability to weaken the integrity of the strongest immune system. And my immune system was no exception. As long as I can remember, my immune system has never been more than average. However, over the last few years, as my detoxing and chelation progressed, this all began to change. In fact, one of the first improvements that I noticed was that I no longer got sick as frequently as I used to. As my mercury levels decreased, my immune system's strength increased dramatically.

Putting all of these factors together—the diluted stomach acid, the lower-than-normal bile volumes, and the weakened immune system—my body seemed to be an irresistible target for opportunistic pathogenic bacteria and parasites. With three systems of defense simultaneously weakened over a significant period of time, the reality of a parasitic invasion seemed to be an inevitable consequence. Of course, this was all more hypothetical speculation. It was just another theory that had been forming in my mind for some time. But this notion of parasites hadn't gained much traction until one particular day while I was on vacation.

I was still keeping a meticulous journal of my experiences, thoughts, theories, and research. It was my custom that when something strange or unexpected happened, I made a special emphasis of this in my journal. One thing that made it into my journal from time to time was an unexpected sensitivity to large amounts of sweets. Being highly sensitive to mercury, MSG, or the halides is one thing—but ordinary sugar? This was strange indeed. I had an incident involving this sensitivity while I was on vacation, and I recorded it in my journal as follows:

*July 8—had sugary food for breakfast (French toast and syrup), lunch (honey on peanut butter and jelly), and a large portion of vanilla ice cream for dinner. Awoke at 3 a.m. with swelling in my right cheek. Stayed up the rest of the night, went for a jog in the early morning, and the swelling had mostly subsided by noon.*

Later on, I went back and did a search through my entire journal. To my surprise, I found several entries that seemed to hint at sensitivity to large amounts of sugary foods. *But why would sugar cause an allergic response?* More research followed. I was looking for any commonalities between sugar sensitivity and the items on my symptom/improvement list that did not have the word "excellent" next to it. I couldn't find any connection between sugar and MSG that satisfied me, but I did find a definite connection between sugar and at least two other symptoms: nausea and rashes.

As strange as it sounds, I found that these two symptoms could quite possibly be connected to a fungal overgrowth. Fungi thrive on sugar, and after bloating themselves on the sweets, the fungi excrete large amounts of toxins as metabolic waste. These wastes can cause a number of health problems, not just nausea and rashes. My personal journal showed several occasions over the past few years where I had an allergic reaction after eating large amounts of sweets.

This information was interesting, even compelling, but I was not yet ready to consider it as evidence. I needed more information, so I continued looking into the research. Eventually I came to a point of saturation with my research findings where it seemed more than just plausible that my remaining symptoms were due in large part to a fungal parasite problem. There could be more parasites involved, but I was fairly certain that at the very least, a pathogenic fungus was involved. As a matter of fact, after looking over my own journal entries and digging even deeper into the data on parasites, I eventually became convinced that my remaining health symptoms were most likely not due to mercury or any other toxin that came from an external source. External toxicity just didn't fit the pattern of my findings, nor did it fit with how I was feeling. I believed all of those external toxins—particularly the mercury—were probably long gone due to the chelation, liver flushes, and thyroid cleansing. No, the connection between high sugar amounts and some of my remaining symptoms pointed to an internal source of toxicity. These symptoms seemed to have been caused by something *living inside of me.*

DETOX MEMOIR

My last adversary in this detoxification battle was organic. It was alive. But was it just a fungal overgrowth, or were there other pathogens like bacteria, protozoa, and even (gasp) worms involved? I did not know the answer to this incredible question...yet.

CHAPTER 39

# From Symbiotic to Parasitic

As I considered the idea of fighting an internal parasite, some of my journal entries—the really weird and inexplicable ones—suddenly began to make perfect sense. Several entries simply did not fit the pattern of other entries. It was almost as if I were fighting an enemy that was moving, responding, and adapting to my various detox protocols. This hadn't made sense to me at the time, because toxic metals like mercury are not alive. Metals don't respond to anything.

However, living things like parasites do. Parasites will respond to external stimuli, especially when the stimuli comes in the form of an attack, which is essentially what a detox protocol is to them. At first, I found this really hard to believe. *Parasites? Isn't that pretty much just a third-world problem where drinking water, swimming water, and waste water are oftentimes the same thing?* But when I got into the actual research on the problem of human parasites, I found an entirely different scenario.

The first thing I found was that I had to demolish many of the preconceived prejudices, stereotypes, and exaggerated notions I had concerning human parasites. For example, most human parasites are microscopic in size, not the three-foot monster tapeworms that can be pulled from a person's mouth. When I was a boy, I heard a story about a person infested with monster tapeworms. That story frightened me for years. No doubt many of us have heard stories like this. Unfortunately, these types of stories create an exaggerated bias and misunderstanding in our minds that is, frankly, difficult to extinguish. The truth of the matter is that most parasites cannot be seen without a microscope. And even with advanced microscopy, parasites are still difficult to detect most of the time. Yes it is true: large parasitic tapeworms do exist, but they are exceedingly rare in comparison to the smaller and vastly more common roundworms and microscopic protozoa.

Besides my misunderstanding of the types of parasites that most commonly afflict humans, I was blithely unaware of the enormous problem of human parasites in the world today. I found research that claimed that approximately half of the world's population is host to a least one type of human parasite! Clearly, parasites are not a third-world problem. They are a worldwide problem. One study conducted in the United States found that over 90 percent of the people examined tested positive for *Enterobius*, commonly known as the pinworm. This was a completely unexpected finding. I had no idea parasites were such a global problem, and I certainly had not thought that they would be a significant issue in any technologically advanced nation.

Misconceptions aside, I did know a few things about human parasites. As designated by the name, a parasite lives off its host and has a deleterious effect on the life of its host. Most parasites produce only a small variety of metabolic waste products, but their waste is exceedingly toxic. According to my research, the most common toxin excreted by parasites is ammonia. While ammonia is the most common toxin, it is not the most powerful. That honor belongs to acetaldehyde, a Group I carcinogen. *Ammonia and acetaldehyde are produced internally in the human system by parasites? I had no idea!* Both of these chemicals are powerful poisons. Ammonia and acetaldehyde can weaken literally every system in the human body—particularly the immune system, which is the final line of defense against parasites.

Ammonia and acetaldehyde can significantly weaken muscles and joints in the body. I could not prove it, but this could have been the point of origin for my bad back so long ago. Years of accumulating parasitically produced ammonia and acetaldehyde (which incidentally, the human body has a very difficult time eliminating) could certainly have been the reason for my chronically painful lower back. The lower back forms the pivot point, or fulcrum, for the entire human body. The muscles that support the lower back could easily have been weakened by years of exposure to acetaldehyde, and this would have put an incredible strain on the lower-back's vertebrae discs.

It was an interesting theory, but not one that I cared to try and prove at the moment. My goal was to detoxify myself. And if I was generating parasitically produced ammonia and acetaldehyde, it was ultimately useless to simply neutralize the effects of these extremely powerful toxins. I needed to attack the source-- the parasites themselves. More research followed, and the picture grew even more grim.

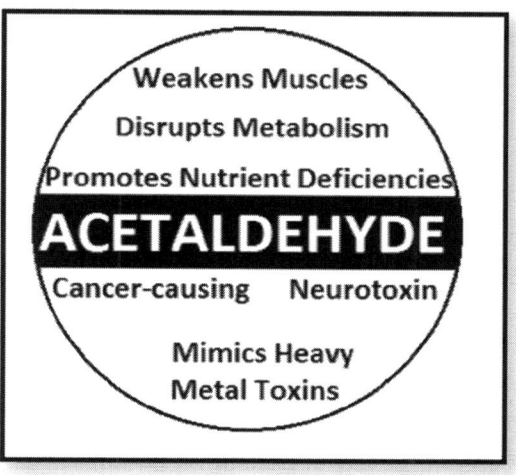

I found that the transmission routes that parasites can take are highly varied. Parasites are able to enter humans via the air, food, water, soil, animals, and other humans. With hundreds of potential parasites so easily able to colonize within humans, any person suffering from toxicity would be extremely vulnerable to a parasitic attack. As I continued delving into the research, I became convinced that if the stomach acid production was compromised, the bile flow restricted, and the immune system weakened, there was a virtual 100 percent guarantee that parasitic infestation would occur.

This was a shocking revelation. I have to admit that when I first considered the possibility of a parasite problem, I thought it was complete nonsense. Now I thought

> When I first considered the possibility of a parasite problem, I thought it was complete nonsense.

differently. How could human parasites thrive in an environment as "clean" as the one in which I lived? The chlorine levels in the municipal water supply alone were sky high, and I was supposed to believe that parasites could survive this, successfully enter my system, and begin to reproduce inside of me? This just seemed too incredible to believe, and yet the data seemed to be pointing to exactly that. Anyone who has a toxicity problem (and that would be most people on the planet) must address the parasite issue, because toxicity inevitably will lead to parasitism of some sort.

I realize this conclusion sounds extreme, but I was taking data and research from highly reputable sources including the World Health Organization, the US Environmental Protection Agency, the Centers for Disease Control, and scholarly peer-reviewed studies. I was simply putting the pieces together. These groups did the difficult research—all I did was connect the dots.

If this all sounds too fantastic, and it did to me at first, let's go back to where I first learned about mercury and consider again the data from the sheep study. In only twenty-nine days of exposure to mercury, the sheep's stomach had accumulated an incredible 929 nanograms of mercury for every gram of stomach tissue. If mercury leaches from the mouth, obviously the stomach will be flooded with this toxic element. Mercury damages or destroys everything in its path, and the stomach's parietal cells are certainly no exception to this. With a decreased ability to manufacture the proper quality and quantity of hydrochloric acid, the human body loses a vital defense mechanism against the influx of parasites found in food and water. *But there are no parasites in my food or water…right?*

This was my thinking, for a while anyway. I am fairly certain it's your thinking as well. Most people consider human parasites to be a third-world problem. But as I researched into this question, many cracks appeared in my logic. Parasites and their eggs are found in all types of foods, particularly produce. Some of our produce comes from third-world countries, and no amount of washing this food in ordinary tap water is going to rinse away all of the parasites or their eggs. Parasites are robust survivors. When they attach their eggs to those grapes, apricots, seeds, or whatever produce you can think of, they are not easily removed. They are also not easily seen. Few people would ever even notice parasitic eggs because many are beyond the range of normal eyesight. The highly contagious *Enterobius*, or pinworm, and the equally contagious hookworm (*Ancylostoma duodenale* and *Necator americanus*) produce translucent eggs that are between 40 and 55 micrometers in length. This is about half the width of a single strand of human hair. Who would ever spot these eggs on food that came from an overseas third-world source? No wonder the World Health Organization estimates that pinworms and hookworms are in the bodies of at least 15 percent of the planet's population.

But parasites are not confined to overseas sources. Some parasites, like the protozoa *Giardia* are found in a majority of US lakes, rivers, and streams. Who hasn't gone swimming in a lake or river without accidentally gulping in at least a little of the water? But let's say you are exceedingly and mind-numbingly cautious in every possible way with your food, drink, air quality, hand washing, hand shaking, swimming, hugging, kissing, and sex. Guess what? You still have a parasite! The yeast Candida is found naturally in the human gut. It exists in perfect symbiosis with the human system until an event that triggers dysbiosis (such as an influx of mercury and/or a dramatic decrease in bile flow), and then the Candida yeast morphs into a parasitic fungus. Now in a fungal state, the Candida will affect virtually every vital area of the human system with its deadly toxic waste products, the most damaging of which is the infamous acetaldehyde.

The point in all of this is that parasites are ubiquitous and unavoidable. There is simply no way to defend against them by external means (hand washing, food preparation, etc.). Freeing oneself from parasites begins and ends through internal means, which I now understood to be stomach acid at full strength, bile flowing at normal volumes, and an uncompromised human immune system. The fact is, parasites thrive exceedingly well in just about every environment we would care to call normal. And if a person's internal defenses of stomach acid, bile flow, and general human immune system were compromised, then that person becomes an easy prey for opportunistic parasites. And after carefully considering all of this data, I believed that person was me.

I assumed that standard modern laboratory tests would easily confirm or deny the presence of parasites, particularly those found in the intestines. This was another false assumption. From what I found in the research, including data from the United States Centers for Disease Control, testing for parasites is easy, but getting accurate results from these tests can be exceedingly difficult. From the parasite's point of view, that makes perfect sense. These little creatures have made a living off the lives of others for millennia. Parasites specialize in operating in the background, just below the threshold of detection. If parasites were easy to detect, they wouldn't be around for long!

The reliability and accuracy of many parasite tests is a paltry 20 percent. Even the CDC recommends sending in three separate stool samples to the lab when testing for intestinal parasites. *Three stool samples? Most people are loath even to do this once. Three times is simply out of the question!* And it gets worse. Studies vary in their ranges, but from all that I could find, approximately half of all human parasitic infections are asymptomatic. If people are not aware that the health problems they have are parasite-related, they will not seek treatment for a cure. No wonder the human parasite problem is such a huge global issue, while at the same time being a vastly underreported one.

While all of this was shocking, it was also quite illuminating. The notion that I had parasites—prolific toxin-generating organisms—in my body for some unknown period of time really gave me some perspective. If this was true, then several of the mysterious journal entries I had written over the past several years made perfect sense. Furthermore, a few events from my past that were not mentioned in my journal also made much more sense now. One such event occurred when I was about fourteen years old.

One summer, some friends and I spent a great deal of time at a local lake. This lake, like many in our area, was rich in organic matter. The water had a dark green hue and the organic matter also made the water somewhat cloudy. But it was summertime, and often it was very hot. This local lake became a favorite place of ours to cool off. Kids who swim and play in lakes frequently, although often unintentionally, take in a few sips of lake water from time to time. I know I did. Anyway, during this particular summer, I experienced some strange digestive and intestinal disturbances. I don't exactly recall all of my symptoms, but I do recall feeling nauseated for about two weeks' time. Normally, like most teenagers, I had a rather ravenous appetite. But during this two-week period, I didn't feel like eating much food at all. I did not see a doctor or seek any medical treatment. In fact, I didn't even tell anyone how I felt. I just wasn't quite myself. Nausea was my main symptom, and food in general just did not agree with me. While this was bothersome, it was not the worst part of my problem. Even to this day, I clearly recall the most irritating and bizarre symptom of this health-challenging situation: I had the most noxious-smelling burps you can imagine. I remember desperately trying to hide this horrid odor from friends and family members. *What is wrong with me? Where did this problem come from? Why do I stink so badly?* To make matters worse, these putrid belches were very frequent and sometimes came on unexpectedly, even violently. I remember one time an erupting belch caught me off guard and simply burst out of my mouth while I was playing a game with some friends. They looked at me with confusion and shock, and when they smelled the rancid air I had just generated, they nearly ran away in disgust. I couldn't blame them. I probably would have done the same thing. My belches smelled like a rotting sulfurous swamp. The nausea and putrid belches lasted for about two weeks, then they mysteriously went away and never returned.

I have always wondered about that stinky burp thing I'd had as a teenager. Well, now that I had done a significant amount of research into human parasites, I think I found my answer. As I said before, my success in detoxing was evidenced by a great many physical and mental improvements, including a greatly enhanced immune system. My immune system now was powerful and robust, but it hadn't always been that way. For most of my life, my immune system was average at best. I was frequently sick with colds, flus, sore throats, and other various ailments. I believe my systemic mercury issues greatly weakened my immune system, my stomach's hydrochloric acid levels, and my liver's bile production. And so, even at a young age, my body was ripe for a parasitic attack.

The protozoa *giardia* is commonly found in freshwater sources around the world. Of all the protozoan parasites, *giardia* has the highest number of reported cases of infection worldwide. This protozoa can easily be transmitted by swallowing lake or river water, particularly water that has a high organic matter content. The most common symptoms of *giardia* infection are digestive and intestinal disturbances, and these are often accompanied by noxious, sulfur-smelling belches. When I was just doing some casual reading concerning *giardia*, I did not see anything unusual, nor did I see any connection to myself until I read about those noxious burps. *Sulfur-smelling burps? That sounds like me way back when I was a teenager!* My symptoms matched perfectly with those who are infected with the *giardia* protozoa.

Of course, this was just another hypothetical conjecture of mine. I had no actual proof that I had been infected with *giardia* as a teenager, but it did make perfect sense with what my symptoms were in those days. By the time I was a teenager, I had several mercury fillings in my mouth. I had very poor eating habits, loved sugary foods, and was frequently sick.

Fast forward a few decades to the present day, and things were very different—for the most part. I was fairly confident that most of the mercury had been chelated out of my body. My immune system was excellent, and my eating habits were very good, with a healthy blend of protein, carbohydrates, fruits, vegetables, and fresh water. But all was not completely well: I still loved sugary foods. In terms of vices, I am sure there are worse ones. Like any vice, there is always something worse. But now that I was considering the very strong possibility of being a host to a potential array of loathsome human parasites, I began to see my love for sweets as fuel for the fire.

I did not consider myself a sugar addict, but I knew reducing my sugar intake would take some serious willpower to do. I've always had a fondness for sweets. As a matter of fact, even as I was making great progress with my detoxing, there were times over the last few years when I intensely craved sweets. Interestingly enough, this was often particularly true after a meal.

Sometimes I would have a bowl of sweetened cereal after dinner to satisfy this craving. I didn't know why; I just knew I liked to eat something sweet after a meal. And I didn't see a problem with it. After all, I was feeling great now, and my current condition was such a vast improvement over how I used to feel, that I didn't see any harm. I felt sure that my detox situation was largely under control. There were just a few minor symptoms left, and considering how far I had come over the past few years, my present situation was fantastic. As a matter of fact, I probably would have ignored the remaining symptoms on my list altogether, were it not for the research I had been doing on human parasites.

Obviously, I had missed something along the way. So I took all of the symptoms that I had dealt with in the last ten years or so and cross-referenced them against intestinal flora problems. In a very short period of time, at least one parasitic suspect emerged that almost perfectly matched my symptoms and conditions. It was the yeast/fungus *Candida Albicans*. I had known about *Candida* for a few years now, but my prior assumptions and focus on the liver and thyroid had kept *Candida* and other parasites on the periphery of my investigation, until now.

As previously stated, *Candida* is a yeast that normally exists in the intestines. It is thought to live symbiotically within the human gut as a food source for intestinal bacteria. But, under certain long-term conditions like bile deprivation or heavy metal toxicity, the *Candida* yeast morphs into a fungus that then migrates out of the intestines and enters the bloodstream. Once in the bloodstream, the fungus will settle opportunistically wherever it can, throughout the body. When I compared my symptoms against *Candida,* it seemed very likely that this is what had happened to me. I'd had both mercury toxicity and bile deprivation for a very long period of time, and I knew that those two factors can make a person ripe for a parasitic invasion. However, I didn't understand just *how* ripe I had become until I really dove into the research.

With a growing certainty about *Candida* and a creeping suspicion that other parasites would also be found living in my system, I began seeing things differently than what I had seen even just a few months earlier. The sugar craving I'd had for years was suddenly understandable. I was feeding billions of extra mouths with every meal I ate. This was an extremely disturbing thought, but I think it was fairly accurate just the same. *Candida* is capable of going almost anywhere in the body, and by producing an incredible seventy-nine different toxins as it feeds, it can be responsible for a huge number of health problems. I really dug into the research on *Candida*, and here are some of the highlights of my findings:

- *Candida* overgrowth can be caused by hormonal birth control pills, antibiotics, high sugar consumption, mercury amalgam fillings, extensive chlorine and fluoride exposure, stress, and decreased bile flow.
- *Candida* can adapt to both oxygen-rich environments (oral thrush, *Candida* in the blood), and oxygen-deprived environments (the intestines). Therefore, it can attack its host literally from head to toe. Because it is considered a facultative anaerobe (which means it is very adaptable), it is very difficult to manage once it is in its fungal form.
- Part of the adaptability of *Candida* is that it is dimorphic. It can exist as both a yeast and a fungus. In its yeast form, it may comprise 3 to 5 percent of the normal intestinal flora, and it is thought to serve as a food source for intestinal bacteria. But once the intestinal pH is altered and the intestinal flora becomes unbalanced, the *Candida* yeast morphs into a fungus, and then it outgrows its intestinal home.
- Candida overgrowth is often linked to gluten sensitivity and celiac disease. The protein that Candida utilizes to attach to the human intestinal wall is extremely similar to the gluten molecule. The human immune system has difficulty in distinguishing between these two molecules, and attacks gluten as if it were a Candida protein.
- Of the seventy-nine different toxins *Candida* can produce as metabolic waste, the most harmful is acetaldehyde, a Group I human

carcinogen (the most dangerous group of cancer-causing substances). Acetaldehyde is the principal chemical behind many, if not most, of the symptoms that accompany *Candida* overgrowth, which may include depression, sleeping problems, irritability, confusion, poor memory, anxiety, leaky gut, obsessive/compulsive behaviors, sexual problems, infertility, dizziness, numbness, sugar cravings, sinusitis, tinnitus, interstitial cystitis, high cholesterol, high blood pressure, acid reflux, rectal itching, excessive difficulty in gaining/losing weight, toenail fungus, hives, prematurely graying hair, allergies, recurring infections like colds and flus, recurring infections of the sinuses and urinary bladder, fibromyalgia, multiple sclerosis, lupus, autism, thyroid imbalances, night sweats, cold feet, muscle and joint pain, endometriosis, chemical sensitivity, dark circles under the eyes, and many other symptoms.

The list of symptoms and conditions caused by *Candida* and its main metabolic waste product, acetaldehyde, was extremely long and troubling. I had personally experienced many of the symptoms caused by this powerful fungus. This was an astonishing find. So many health problems caused by a single organism. I was fairly certain I'd played host to the *giardia* protozoa as a teenager, and since there were well over 100 common parasites that could incubate inside humans, I was probably playing host to a literal zoo of other harmful parasitic organisms. By sheer probability alone, most of these uninvited guests were microscopic in size. But embedded deep in the back of my mind was that old fear that I desperately tried to suppress. *Oh please don't let there be any monster-sized tapeworms living inside of me!*

Irrational fears aside, it was a proven fact that I had *Candida* because *Candida* is in everyone. It was also a proven fact that the *Candida* yeast can morph into a fungus if the human host has toxicity issues, which I did. It was also a proven fact that *Candida* fungus produces seventy-nine toxic chemicals as a waste product, including acetaldehyde. This was all bad news, and to make matters even worse, most parasites, including *Candida*, feed on sugar. We give our *Candida* sugar, and it gives us poison. Talk about a bad exchange.

In spite of these challenges, there were many factors that were presently working in my favor. Detoxing for several years now had rewarded me with a powerful and robust immune system and this did not bode well for any opportunistic parasites. I was also confident that my thyroid and liver were functioning at, or nearly at, maximum efficiency. This would mean that bile was flowing at normal volumes and at a fully concentrated strength. This would cause my intestines to be a fairly inhospitable place for intestinal parasites, including the *Candida* fungus.

But parasites are tenacious, and they are exceptionally adept at evading detection. So I designed a comprehensive, all-natural protocol to gently but firmly remove any existing parasites. I felt intuitively that I was at the end of my detox journey, and I wasn't going to take any chances with how I went about implementing these last few steps. If there were parasites living in my system, they wouldn't be there for much longer. They had to go.

Getting rid of microscopic parasites is one thing, but getting rid of *Candida* was a bit trickier. *Candida* is in everyone. We're born with it, and we'll die with it. *Candida* is an important part of a normal person's intestinal flora, and there was no way to get rid of it. So what I needed to do was to find a way to quickly and efficiently eliminate the fungal roots and branches (called hyphae) that were possibly running throughout my body. Then I could coerce the *Candida* back into its yeast form in the intestines. In short, I needed to find a way to put the fungal monster back into its cage.

Since it was by far the most common of all human parasites and because many of my symptoms matched very closely with *Candida* fungal overgrowth, I put most of my focus on the *Candida* issue first. Researching *Candida* fungal overgrowth was surprisingly easy. There is a tremendous amount of information concerning *Candida* health-related problems on the web. I'd had no idea the *Candida* fungus condition was such a huge issue worldwide. What I really found most interesting, though, was the chemistry of acetaldehyde, the most harmful of *Candida's* metabolic wastes.

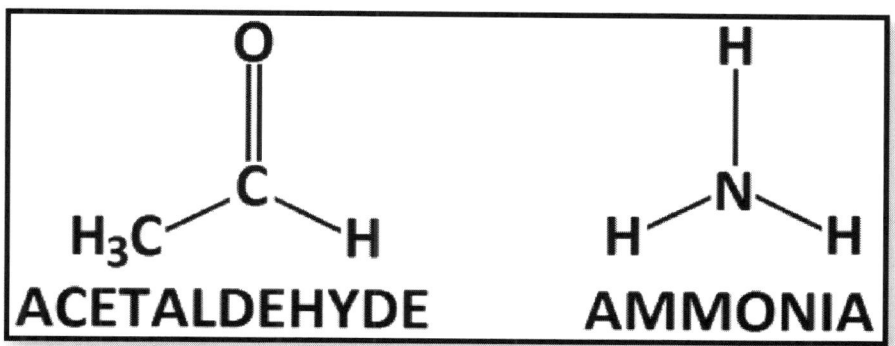

As has already been mentioned, the two most damaging chemicals that human parasites produce as waste products are acetaldehyde and ammonia. Both of these chemicals are powerful toxins, and it amazed me that these very small molecules could cause such a large variety of health problems. Ammonia is produced naturally by all of the tissues in the human body. Since ammonia is highly toxic, the body closely monitors ammonia amounts and deliberately keeps its concentrations in the blood at extremely low levels. Most of our ammonia is transformed by the liver into a substance called urea. Urea is later eliminated by the body mainly as urine via the kidneys. A small percentage of it is eliminated through human sweat. Since most parasites produce ammonia as a waste product, it seemed logical that a parasite's presence would put additional stress on the liver, since it would have to process more ammonia into urea.

Further increasing the stress on the liver was the presence of the highly toxic acetaldehyde. One of the more interesting aspects of this toxin—and one of the main reasons it caught my attention—is that acetaldehyde behaves chemically as if it were a metal. This is unusual. There is no metal atom found in the acetaldehyde molecule. However, because it behaves as a metal, acetaldehyde has a strong affinity for sulfur, selenium, and iodine, the three elements that are absolutely essential for the body's detoxification system. Once again, I had found a powerful chemical that, like mercury, was capable of disarming the body's own natural detox mechanisms. Mercury and acetaldehyde together were indeed a deadly duo. And, on top of all of this, I found data that pointed to acetaldehyde as being the main culprit for my high sensitivity to MSG—monosodium glutamate. This was one question that I found no satisfactory answer for over the last eleven years, until now. While I knew that acetaldehyde has been linked to "leaky gut" syndrome, I did not know that one of the body's main defenses against this attack on the integrity of the intestinal wall was to release generous amounts of the amino acid glutamine. Acetaldehyde tries to punch holes in the intestinal walls, and the body responds by releasing glutamine to prevent this. This was all a fact. My theory was simply this: a person with serious Candida issues would be producing huge amounts of glutamine in order to mitigate the acetaldehyde attack. MSG is a form of highly concentrated glutamine, and any exposure to this much glutamine all at once might provoke an allergic reaction. MSG in foods in conjunction with already high amounts of glutamine in the intestines pushes the body too far. It cannot possibly process that much glutamine in such a short period of time. So the body responds to this glutamine overload with swelling, hives, and about 12 hours of misery. At least, this was my body's response to a glutamine overdose. Well, it was an interesting theory, and once again it was one that I could not prove. But it did explain a major question that I had been wrestling with for over a decade.

With all of these findings, I was certain that my entire detox investigation had finally come full circle. I was sure I now knew the source of my toxicity, and I had a fairly comprehensive understanding of the biochemical mechanisms involved. It had taken eleven years to get here, but I was confident that I had finally arrived at the endpoint.

As I have already stated, I believe the source of my problems began before I drew my first breath. My body was literally built with a fetal blood supply that was contaminated with mercury metal. Later on, I was nursed with mercury-laced milk as an infant. Then I was given mercury metal in my vaccinations as a toddler. And as an 8 or 9 year old boy, I was given my first mercury amalgam filling. All of this toxic mercury inflicted havoc on my liver, thyroid, and intestines. Yes, there were other areas that were damaged, but these three areas were essentially my "detox control center." Once these three areas were compromised, there was no hope of my body being able to fight this toxic battle and win. Years passed, and I continued to accumulate mercury metal that leached from my fillings. My thyroid, already weakened by years of mercury exposure, was further compromised by the halogens in tap water (fluorine and chlorine) and in certain foods (bromine). Over time, these toxins weakened my thyroid to the point that it could no longer produce the thyroid hormone thyroxin in sufficient amounts. This directly led to the formation of gallstones in the liver. These stones prevented my already toxic liver from producing the half liter of vital bile it should have been supplying to the intestines on a daily basis. This lack of normal bile flow eventually affected the intestinal pH and opened up the door to a potential plethora of parasites. These parasites produced a variety of toxins as metabolic wastes, with acetaldehyde and ammonia being the principal destructive agents.

And that, dear reader, is the summary of my terrible toxic drama. Years ago, I had felt that my body was telling me that I was being poisoned. It turns out that feeling was correct. Mercury, ammonia, acetaldehyde, fluorine, chlorine, and bromine are all poisons. These were the sinister six chemicals that were responsible for the decline of my health.

# Chapter 40

# Welcome to Your Life

After eleven long years, I had finally found the remaining missing pieces to my detox puzzle. This finding gave me an amazing sense of closure and perspective. Physically, I felt fantastic. Knowing the actual causes of my problems gave me an overwhelming sense of relief and gratitude. And there was still more good news. I was fairly confident that four out of the six chemicals were already effectively mitigated or removed with the chelation, liver flushes, and thyroid boosters. The swelling and hives were long gone, and so I hardly ever used my activated charcoal anymore. I continued to do liver flushes once or twice per year on a sort of ongoing maintenance schedule. I continued to take my thyroid boosters daily, but only at minimum level dosages, and of course, I continued to take my normal high-potency multivitamins. I felt that these would all help my body with the Candida problem and its main henchman, acetaldehyde.

This was all very good, but there was still the question of the other human parasites that had potentially stolen their way into my body back when my immune system, bile flow amounts, and stomach acid production was so greatly compromised. What was I to do about this potential problem?

More research followed. Over a fairly short period of time, I developed a strategy for parasite removal. The strategy was elegantly simple. It had only three facets.

1. Eliminate the parasites' hiding places.
2. Focus primarily on the *Candida* issue.
3. Use only natural substances that could also be used as food.

With respect to the first facet of my protocol, I knew that well over a hundred different species of parasites could colonize within humans. It didn't make any sense to try to chase down and destroy each and every type of these uninvited guests. Parasites are hardy survivors. They specialize in evading detection. They have an incredible ability to adapt to their environment, particularly when that environment becomes hostile to their existence. Rather than explore each and every potential species, I decided to implement a more practical solution. I would find a way to demolish the parasites' hiding places; then they would be exposed to the body's own natural mechanisms like full-strength bile, healthy levels of normal intestinal flora, and normal concentrations of acid in the stomach. This would allow these natural mechanisms to do what they were designed to do, and the parasites would be vanquished. This is how animal species throughout the world are made extinct. Destroy the habitat first, and eventually the animals are history. But habitat destruction was just one part of my simple plan for eliminating parasites.

The second part of my strategy was to focus on *Candida*. It was the one parasite that I was certain I had, because everyone has it. The real question was, had the *Candida* yeast morphed into its fungal form? I was fairly certain that it had because of how closely my symptoms matched those of *Candida* fungal overgrowth. Furthermore, the former state of my body had been ripe for an influx of parasitic invaders. I was convinced that if indeed there was a *Candida* fungal problem and my chosen protocol could successfully remove or reduce a fungus, it would most likely remove or reduce the populations of the other parasites as well.

I dove into mainstream medicine's research on *Candida* fungal removal, but I was not optimistic I would find much that I could actually use. I realize this sounds terribly pessimistic, but I had learned some very hard lessons over the last decade, and so I was extremely wary of any pharmaceutical cure-all. Despite my bias and skepticism, I wanted to know what was commonly used by medical practitioners for this problem. Not surprisingly, the most common form of treatment for *Candida* overgrowth is an array of prescription antifungal medications. I didn't have to dig too deeply to find that this treatment has only limited success. And this observation did not come from me. It came from both within and without the mainstream medical community. The recurring theme was that antifungals are typically effective only in the short term and with non-systemic conditions.

As prescription medications, antifungals carry powerful and undesirable side effects, particularly over a long-term use. And once the antifungal treatment has concluded, *Candida* eventually returns, often in a more powerful and aggressive form. This made sense to me. According to both the liver toxicity cycle and the detox triangle, unless normal bile volumes are released into the intestine, a normal intestinal environment has not been reestablished. In a very real sense, the intestines are still *Candida* friendly. Without normal bile volumes flowing through the intestines, it is impossible for the normal pH balance to be reestablished.

A person taking antifungal medication will experience some relief, temporarily. The drugs do work, but only for a limited period of time. Once the antifungal drugs are discontinued, *Candida* comes out of its various hiding places and it is back in business. Taking another round of antifungal medication is what many people do, only to see the same thing happen again later on, worsening the person's overall condition. But this worsening of a person's condition was not only due to the return of the fungus, but also due to the horrid side effects that accompany nearly all prescription medications.

While my findings on the negative aspects of prescription antifungal medications were not surprising, I did find one aspect that was somewhat illuminating. The actual reasons for the side effects. *Why do anti-fungal medications have side effects?* This was a very good question. A main component of the fungal cellular membrane is a chemical called *ergosterol*. Human cells do not have ergosterol. Neither do animals. As a matter of fact, I could not find any plant species that carried the ergosterol molecule. But both plants, animals, and humans

> Why do anti-fungal medications have side effects?

produce something similar to ergosterol in their bodies. This molecule is called *cholesterol*, and herein lies the difficulty. Shown here are molecular models of cholesterol and ergosterol. If you have difficulty in distinguishing the differences between these two molecules, you are not alone. Apparently, most of the medications used to treat fungal overgrowth have this same difficulty.

**ERGOSTEROL**

**CHOLESTEROL**

And that is exactly the point. The confusion in distinguishing between friend and foe is one reason that antifungals have that all-too-typical list of negative side effects. They range from the mild (nausea, headaches, rashes) to the severe (kidney damage, heart damage, liver failure), depending on the individual. From all I could find, taking an antifungal was very similar to taking an antibiotic. Antibiotics wipe out both helpful and harmful bacteria with equally destructive force. Antifungals are similar, only the antifungal attacks good cells due to their cholesterol content, along with the bad cells with their ergosterol content.

Obviously I did not want to go this route. My goal from the very beginning had been to find and utilize protocols that did not involve prescription medications. The rather lengthy list of side effects attached to the various antifungals only solidified my resolve in this matter. But if taking prescription antifungal medication was not an option, what other options were there for eliminating *Candida*?

I did a significant amount of research on the so-called *Candida* starvation diets, but ultimately decided they would not work for me. One, I wasn't convinced that any starvation diet would really affect the *Candida*—but it would certainly affect me. *Candida* would outlive and outlast me, no matter how much, or how little, sugar I consumed. Limiting my sugar intake was something I knew I needed to do, but to try and starve the Candida to death was not going to work. When parasites like Candida find themselves in a hostile environment, or one that is lacking in food, they don't die. They simply retreat into a spore form and remain dormant until more favorable conditions return. When those conditions reappear, such as a person coming off a *Candida* starvation diet or discontinuing the prescription antifungal drug, the parasite reemerges and wreaks havoc once again. Furthermore, these diets didn't even sound healthy to me. They were too extreme and too restrictive. I wasn't about to eat only brown rice and raw vegetables for the next couple of years. I felt I had a much simpler answer. I would make sure normal concentrations of stomach acid and bile were restored and that my immune system was near or at full strength. Then I would destroy the parasite's habitat and let the body do the rest. If I could eliminate the hiding places in my high state of health, I could destroy whole populations of parasites. It really was that simple.

The next question to be explored was where the human parasites actually hid. I was fairly confident at this point that I already knew the answer. I had accumulated so much information about detoxing over the last eleven years, I had seen a great deal of repetition in the research. Many of the same studies and stories reappeared again and again. At this point in my journey, the quest wasn't so much about finding the answers as it was about asking the right questions.

I knew that parasites could be found anywhere in a body that has weakened stomach acid production, reduced bile flow, and a seriously compromised immune system. Once these three factors were restored to their normally functioning levels, the last holdout for the parasites had to be in the very substance generated by the body to protect itself from a parasite's toxic waste: the mucus membranes.

The key to the hidden habitat mystery was actually just simple mucus. *Why mucus?* It is well known that *Candida* and other parasites produce large amounts of toxic chemical waste products. These chemicals are extremely irritating to the internal tissues of the body. As a response to the presence of these highly irritating chemicals, the body produces generous amounts of mucus to protect these sensitive tissues. But mucus also provides a measure of protection for many of the parasites themselves, particularly within the digestive system. So in a somewhat paradoxical way, the same substance that protects the human body from parasitically produced metabolic wastes also protects the parasites from the body's parasite-destroying agents. The agents that were designed to destroy things like parasites were again, stomach acid, bile, and the human immune system. Mucus membranes are found almost everywhere in the body. Therefore, parasites could also be found nearly everywhere. This is why breaking down the excess mucus throughout the digestive system is so important. And this is one of the many roles of stomach acid and bile.

But here is the interesting thing: I felt that this was already working inside of me, and I had some fairly compelling evidence in support of this. I felt great almost all of the time now. The last few health symptoms that I still had to deal with were actually quite minor, especially compared to what they had been before. My thinking was clear, my memory was sharp, my strength and stamina were outstanding, and I had energy to burn. And I was doing this all on only one or two meals a day. As I have already mentioned, I had been eating significantly less food these past few years. This naturally caused my waistline to shrink. But I didn't lose any overall weight. My weight sort of just shifted from my belly to my chest and shoulders. Furthermore, I didn't feel the urgent need for food (or sweets) like I used to have. Yes, I still enjoyed sweets. But I didn't crave them. The same was true for food in general. One or two meals easily provided all that I required to keep going. I believed the reason for this body upgrade was my clean and clear thyroid. Once my thyroid was clean from the toxins that had polluted it, my metabolism vastly improved, and I processed food far more efficiently than I had before.

But something else was going on as well. Not eating as much but still continuing on with my same weight meant that the absorption levels of the food that I did eat must have enormously improved. It was the only thing that made sense to me. This notion was supported by the use of my regular multivitamins, particularly my vitamin C supplement. I seemed to get far greater benefit from these supplements now than I ever had before. But the food and the vitamins had not changed. I was the one that had changed. And I credited these changes to a greatly enhanced thyroid and a cleaned up digestive system that had plenty of healthy intestinal flora and very little excess mucus. However, apparently not all of the excess mucus had been burned away, because I still had a few lingering symptoms, and I reasoned that these may have been due to parasites.

Did I have any proof for all of this speculation? No. As a matter of fact, I wasn't even sure I had a parasite problem to begin with. It just seemed logical. Instinctively I felt I was on the right path. But I had no actual proof to back up my theories. But I had been doing this detox thing for so long now that, as unscientific as this sounds, I just knew I was going in the right direction. I knew my body was doing great, but I also felt that I could get it to an even higher level of health and efficiency. It just needed a little extra help.

So, as I have already mentioned, the parasite-removal protocol that I formulated was extremely simple. The goal was to eliminate or at least reduce the number of parasite hiding places. I believed those were areas that contained excess mucus. And if there were nothing but *Candida* fungi in those areas, that would be more than enough. I felt that reducing the fungal population even a little, would bring positive benefits to my health because any reduction of acetaldehyde exposure would be highly beneficial. And I was determined to use only food to do this. No medications or prescriptions were required for my final protocol. The reason for this was actually quite simple. If you eliminate medical prescriptions as a curative measure, what else is left to bring about healing? *Food. It had to be food.* But it couldn't be just any type of food. If the solution was just regular food, my problems would have spontaneously resolved themselves years ago. No, I needed foods that were available in their highest concentrations; foods with well-known antibacterial and antifungal properties. That's what I was going to use to solve this final health mystery.

Perhaps you have already guessed what I am referring to. If you are thinking of essential oils and healing herbs, you are correct. Way back at the beginning of my journey, I had done some research and then dabbled with essential oils and herbs, but I eventually abandoned the oils and herbs because I seemed to have gotten little if any use out of them. Now with a cleaned up liver, thyroid, and intestinal system, I was fairly confident that this second exploration into essential oils and healing herbs would bring vastly different results. And I was not disappointed.

I decided to use three essential oils: oil of oregano, cinnamon bark oil, and peppermint oil. As was my long-time custom, I began with very small daily doses just to see how I would react. I focused most of my attention on the oil of oregano because it had the most powerful antifungal and antibacterial properties of the three. Starting with just a few drops daily, I gradually increased my dosage over time in search of an upper limit of tolerance. I had done this before with other supplements, most notably the nascent iodine, and I'd found this to be the best way to introduce a new supplement into the daily regimen. After just a few days of gradually increasing the oil, I got a Herxheimer reaction—some slight facial swelling. This was actually very good news. It told me that I was on the right track. Something nasty must have been dying off on the inside of me. Was it bacterial or fungal in makeup? I did not know. But something good was happening, so I increased my dosage again, carefully trying to stay aggressive but not to the point of provoking any more Herxheimer reactions.

After just a few weeks of taking the oregano oil, I began to see small improvements—even more energy, sleeping more soundly through the night, and just a better overall feeling of wellness. After a few months of this, I found that the underarm rashes that I had tolerated for years were gone! Furthermore, other little annoyances like aching in the joints and heavy legs, which I had formerly attributed to aging, had greatly diminished. I also found that my MSG sensitivity seemed to have decreased even more. I never did binge on foods that I knew had MSG as a test for this, but I did eat moderate portions of foods that contained MSG, and I had no allergic reaction. This was incredible! The only conclusion I could draw from all of this was that these symptoms had to be tied to some sort of parasite and its production of toxic waste products like acetaldehyde and ammonia. So, if you reduce parasite counts via essential oils—in my case, a high-quality oil of oregano, cinnamon, and peppermint—you will reduce the internally produced toxins by those parasites.

All this was very good, but still I wasn't satisfied with this rate of progress. *What could I do to make sure my naturally produced bile and the essential oils I was supplementing with got into even closer contact with the tissues—particularly those that line the intestinal tract?* Sticking with the notion that the body produces excess amounts of mucus to protect against internally produced toxins, I wondered if it was possible to mechanically scrape my digestive system, internally, to get rid of any excess mucus. If this could be done, then my normally produced bile and the essential oils would have an even greater contact with key tissues, and my already excellent progress would only increase. After doing a bit more research, I discovered a method that farmers use around the world to help their livestock stay parasite-free. *It was time to eat a little dirt.*

Well, that's what I thought when I first read about using food-grade diatomaceous earth. I found plenty of information supporting the use of this material for parasite elimination. "What? You mean eating diatomaceous earth can scrape my intestines clean of excess mucus and any lingering parasites?" *Yes, that's exactly what I mean.* Diatomaceous earth (DE) has a long history of being used for precisely this purpose. DE is not exactly dirt, but it can be safely used as a food nutrient as long as it is of food-grade quality. DE contains several important minerals, the most important of which is silicon. While these minerals were useful to anyone, the reason I wanted to take DE was not for what it could do for me chemically, but mechanically.

DE is an exceptionally fine powder. It is also exceedingly hard. This makes DE a powerful abrasive, and microscopic parasites have no defense against it. They are totally vulnerable to this almost completely inert substance. And better still, there is no way for them to adapt to its presence in the human body, because it wouldn't be chemistry that was killing them; it was physics. From all I found in the research, adding DE to livestock feed is a powerfully efficient and logically cost-effective tool that farmers use to keep their livestock's digestive systems parasite-free.

Well, if it was good enough for the cows and pigs, it was good enough for me.

As usual, I began with small amounts and worked my way up. After only a week, I was taking about two tablespoons of food-grade DE daily. Mixed with water, it tasted like a combination of chalk and seawater. But mixed with juice, it had very little taste at all. It still had a bit of a chalky texture, but the results were well worth the effort. After only a few days at this dosage, I found that the solid waste I was producing mirrored the results that I had gotten years ago when I first started making real progress with expelling heavy metals from my body. The DE supplement appeared to be doing its job rather nicely. Here is a portion of my journal entry at this time:

*Solid waste is extremely pungent, sticky, and very heavy. Have no idea what is in it, but it is waste in a very real sense.*

Looking back, I suppose it would have been a good idea to take a stool sample of this stinky sticky mass and send it off to the lab. But research had already shown me that the accuracy of parasite testing in stool samples is abysmally low. And like most people, taking a stool sample was inherently repugnant. I just could not bring myself to do much more than give the solid waste a passing backward glance before I flushed it down. Even with these brief backward glances, I never saw anything unusual or dramatic like a gigantic fluke or the corpse of a monster-sized tapeworm. The vast majority of parasites are microscopic in size, so any cursory visual inspection was doubly useless.

The protocol of taking essential oils and food-grade diatomaceous earth went on for several months. During this time I also supplemented with some capsules that were filled with a variety of healing herbs specifically formulated to kill any internal parasite (protozoa, fungal, or bacterial), but leave the natural, healthy bacterial flora unharmed. I took this rather broad spectrum approach to my potential parasite problem because I wasn't taking any chances. I knew I was at the end of my detox journey, and if there was a parasite problem, I wanted to end it quickly. I needed to hit the parasites with everything I could think of in the arsenal that was available to me. Bile at full strength. Fully concentrated stomach acid. Nascent iodine and multivitamin and mineral supplementation. Essential oils. Parasite-killing herbs. Food-grade diatomaceous earth. This went on for about six months. When it was all over, what did I have? How had I changed?

Well, to begin with, I never did have any of those dramatic, over-the-top, "Oh yuck…take a look at what just came out of me" moments in the bathroom. Thankfully, there was no drama with my parasite cleanse. I never saw anything unusual, and I was very glad for that. However, just because I didn't see anything weird come out of me doesn't mean that something weird didn't. I think it did; it was just too small to see.

I experienced a few very interesting improvements over the course of my six months or so of parasite cleansing. One of the first things I noticed was that I didn't have the sugar cravings anywhere near what I used to have. After my six-month parasite cleanse, my after-dinner sugar cravings were almost completely gone. As a matter of fact, some of the high-sugar foods that I used to eat or drink in the past now slightly nauseated me. Most sweets just seemed to taste too sweet. I had always loved peanut butter and jelly sandwiches. I used to heap on the jelly in the old days because I loved the sweetness of it. I couldn't do that anymore. I still enjoyed my peanut butter and jelly, but only if I used a sparse amount of jelly. That was all I needed to have the perfect sandwich.

I found this to be true with all of my old favorite sweet foods—cakes, pies, cookies, whatever. It was also true with sweet-tasting drinks. I couldn't even drink an entire can of soda any longer. It just seemed far too sweet to even enjoy. Drinking soda was now more like a punishment. This was truly an astonishing change. Years earlier, I used to drink soda like it was water—literally. Now I could hardly tolerate it.

But there is more. Food itself tasted differently now. Junk food now tasted like recycled waste. This was fine, because I really didn't need to eat that sort of thing anyway. I didn't need it, and now I didn't want it, so it was really the perfect arrangement. Meanwhile, good, high-quality food tasted absolutely amazing. In fact, good food tasted better to me now than it had in maybe a decade or two. It's very hard to explain really. It was almost as if my taste buds had reawakened. Food now reminded me of what it was like back when I was much younger. I really looked forward to a good meal, because it was so incredibly satisfying. And perhaps best of all, most foods didn't carry any awful aftertaste. I rarely experienced that post-meal bloated feeling anymore. And if I did get that sour stomach feeling after a meal, taking a few drops of one of the essential oils usually made my stomach purr like a kitten.

I theorized that the reason for all of this improvement was due to several changes that were now working synergistically. A cleaned-up thyroid now allowed my metabolism to operate at its maximum efficiency. My cleaned-up liver had been producing fully concentrated bile for some time now. This bile, in conjunction with the essential oils, food-grade diatomaceous earth, and healing herbs had drastically decreased the parasite population throughout my system. This directly led to a sharp reduction in parasite production of ammonia and acetaldehyde, and that led to my achieving an even greater level of health and wellness.

Even though I was very skeptical at first concerning the idea of human parasites and their connection to toxicity, I no longer had any doubts. I was now certain that decreasing the parasite count in my system was the final fix that was required. My metabolic, digestive, and immune systems were now operating at levels of efficiency that I believe I had never experienced before.

One of my principal goals when I first started this detox was to find some way to restore all of those years that were lost due to ill health. Now at the end of my journey, after twelve years of trials and testing, I truly felt I had regained all of those lost years. But I had gained more. I could see very clearly that now my children were experiencing the benefits of my long journey too. They were in excellent health, and full of life. The chain of mercury toxicity transmission that had been spanning the generations in my family, had been broken at last.

# Epilogue

Detoxing has become somewhat of a fashionable term lately. When I first started my journey over twelve years ago, I don't even recall hearing the term, much less knowing what it meant. Now we hear about detoxing all of the time. Because I spent a great deal of time and energy researching and testing various detox theories and protocols, I am often asked questions concerning this now rather trendy topic.

"If I wanted to do a detox, what would you suggest is the single most important thing that I should do?" This question is a very simple one, and yet in many ways it is a difficult one to answer. My research and findings contradicted many of the conventional teachings and dictums from mainstream medicine and from the scientific community. And over the last seven years, I had compiled quite a list of unconventional ideas and protocols.

Having said all of this, when I am asked this question, I usually respond by saying that the best detox should focus not so much on putting expensive chemicals into your body, but on taking the inexpensive chemicals out.

I know from experience that when people feel that they are ready to do a detox, their approach is usually very much the same that mine was back at the beginning of my journey. People want to take a pill or powder; a gel, a cream, or an essential oil; or go on an incredibly restrictive diet. They might also choose to go the prescription route, particularly when they are facing what they believe to be a *Candida* fungal overgrowth.

I believe the single best thing a person can do to detox themselves is not to put something new into their system, but to take something old out. Take out those old mercury fillings. Remove the blockage from your liver with regular liver flushes. Chelate out the mercury and halogens that have crippled your thyroid function by using simple yet powerful supplements like nascent iodine, selenium, and zinc. Scrape from the intestines the moldy old mucus that both hinders intestinal performance and harbors a plethora of pathogens. In the final analysis, removing the old toxins is what led to most of my healing, not the taking in of copious and oftentimes expensive supplements.

A friend of mine asked me recently how a person can know whether they need to detox or not. Without hesitation, I replied that all people need to detox periodically, because we all live in a toxic world. There are toxins in the food we eat, the water we drink, and the air we breathe. So naturally we all need to detox ourselves from these chemicals from time to time.

"Yes, I understand this," my friend replied. "But my patients do not. Could you come up with an idea, maybe a survey of some sort that would help people determine if they need to detox or not?"

I confess that I could not think of anything that could help convince people to do a detox, apart from simply telling my own story and encouraging them to do the research for themselves.

And that is what I have done here. Now you know my detox story. Many years ago I was dreadfully sick; now I am well. My story here contains most of the reasons and details of how I did it. I said at the very beginning that this book would *not* change your life. God can change your life. You can change your life. And you can start this change, towards a bright and vibrant future, today.

# Acknowledgments

I would like to thank several people for assisting with the content and writing of this book. First of all, I need to give special thanks to my family and close friends who heard me say countless times, "I have this new theory that I want to tell you about." Thank you for not rolling your eyes too many times when I said something concerning my latest evolving theory. Special thanks to my very talented editors and readers: Carrie Bost, Sue Houston, Christopher Moore, Jules Dorais, Jennifer Olivier, Kevin Whitted, Barb Thorpe, and the CreateSpace editorial team. Thanks also to Joel Holsinger, Mwita Chacha, and Riann Sundt for their artistic expertise.

I would like to acknowledge the pioneering work of Dr. Weston Price, a true visionary far ahead of his time, whose work provided a great deal of inspiration for this book. Special thanks to Mr. John Altic, Dr. Alan Greenberg, Dr. Hal Huggins, Dr. Michael Margolis, Dr. Kevin Wall, Dr. George Georgiou, Dr. David Brownstein, Dr. Andy Cutler, and Dr. Jay Danto. The research and insights from these highly talented health professionals provided this memoir with a great deal of balance and perspective. Special thanks to family and friends who contributed inspiration and sometimes their hair samples—including Dr. Gig Dorais, Mary Ann Rivers, Dena Wall, Dawn Gregory, Jill Butler Gregory, Steve Currier, Sarah House White, Ann Biberdorf Smith, Ashley Johnston, and Cody Bishop. A special thanks to Doug Fougnies and Lance Casillas, who provided me with excellent confirming data. Thanks also to Mr. Joe Johnston and Mrs. Kelly Young, who were the first two people to see credibility in my research. Finally, I would like to acknowledge my mother, the late Mary M. Dorais. My mother died long before this book came to fruition, but in so many ways she paved the way for this work with her inquisitive mind and unyielding quest for scientific truth.

# References

**Chapter 6: Asking the Right Questions**

Jacob, S., Lawrence, R. & Zucker, M. (1999). *The Miracle of MSM: The Natural Solution for Pain.* New York, NY: Berkley Books.

Blaylock, R. (1997). *Excitotoxins—The Taste that Kills.* Albuquerque, NM: Health Press NA Inc.

**Chapter 8: By Any Other Name**

MSG Aliases Exposed. (2011). Retrieved from http://www.truthinlabeling.org/MSG.Aliases.Exposed.htm

**Chapter 11: Too Much Trust**

Huggins, H. (1993). *It's All in Your Head—The Link Between Mercury Amalgam and Illness.* New York, NY: Penguin Putnam.

Levy, T. & Huggins, H. (1999). *Uniformed Consent—The Hidden Dangers in Dental Care.* Newburyport, MS: Hampton Publishing.

Windham, B. (2001). Mercury exposure levels from amalgam dental fillings; documentation of mechanisms by which mercury causes over 40 chronic health conditions; results of replacement of amalgam fillings; and occupational effects on dental staff. Retrieved from http://www.fda.gov/ohrms/dockets/dailys/02/Sep02/091602/80027dde.pdf

## Chapter 12: Frailty, Thy Name Is Mercury

Koral, Stephen M., (2005). The scientific case against amalgam. *International Academy of Oral Medicine & Toxicology.* Retrieved from http://iaomt.org/wp-content/uploads/The-Case-Against-Amalgam.pdf

Siegel, S., Stratton, L., Bender, B., & Gutierrez, R. (2003) Mercury exposé: the world's toxic time bomb. Prepared for the 22nd United Nations Environment Programme, Nairobi. Retrieved from http://www.ban.org/Ban-Hg-Wg/Mercury.ToxicTimeBomb.Final.PDF

United States Department of Health and Human Services (1999). Public Health Statement: Mercury. Cas#: 7439-97-6. Washington D.C. Government Printing Office. Retrieved from http://www.atsdr.cdc.gov/ToxProfiles/tp46-c1-b.pdf

United States Environmental Protection Agency (1997). Mercury study report to Congress vol. 5: health effects of mercury and mercury compounds. Washington D.C. Government Printing Office. Retrieved from http://www.epa.gov/ttn/oarpg/t3/reports/volume5.pdf

United States Food and Drug Administration (2009). Dental devices: classification of dental amalgam, reclassification of dental mercury, designation of special controls for dental amalgam, mercury, and amalgam alloy. Food and Drug Administration, Dept. of Health and Human Services. Retrieved from

# REFERENCES

http://www.fda.gov/downloads/medicaldevices/productsandmedicalprocedures/dentalproducts/dentalamalgam/ucm174024.pdf

## Chapter 13: Skeptical Yet?

Sayer, G., Nelson, J., and Colwell, R. (1975). Role of bacteria in bioaccumulation of mercury in the oyster Crassostrea virginica. Applied Microbiology, 30 (1), 91-96. Retrieved from http://www.ncbi.nlm.nih.gov/pmc/articles/PMC187121/

## Chapter 14: Plotting a Course

United States Environmental Protection Agency (2013). Mercury in dental amalgam. Retrieved from http://www.epa.gov/hg/dentalamalgam.html

Cutler, A. (1999). *Amalgam Illness, Diagnosis and Treatment: What You Can Do to Get Better, How Your Doctor Can Help.* Sammamish, WA: Andrew Hall Cutler Publishing.

Cutler, A. (1999). *Hair Test Interpretation: Finding Hidden Toxicities.* Noamalgam.com.

## Chapter 15: Taking that First Step

Kuligowski, J. & Halperin, K. (1992). Stainless steel cookware as a significant source of nickel, chromium, and iron. *Archives of Environmental Contamination and Toxicology*, 23, 211-215. Retrieved from http://link.springer.com/article/10.1007/BF00212277#page-1

## Chapter 19: The Terrifying Theoretical Leap

Kennedy, D. (2011). US FDA hearings on amalgam safety. Retrieved from https://www.youtube.com/watch?v=jK2Uy49Z6CA and https://www.youtube.com/watch?v=pUcSrOycSME

American Dental Association Council on Scientific Affairs (2010). Literature review: dental amalgam fillings and health effects. Retrieved from http://www.ada.org/en/member-center/oral-health-topics/amalgam

## Chapter 21: Breaking Through

Georgiou, G. (2007). Flushing gallstones naturally. Retrieved from http://www.collegenaturalmedicine.com/images/LBA/liver%20cleansing%202007.pdf

## Chapter 22: The New Plan

Brody, J. (1995, May 31). Personal health; gallbladder surgery is easier. Is it too common? *The New York Times*. Retrieved from http://www.nytimes.com/1995/05/31/us/personal-health-gallbladder-surgery-is-easier-is-it-too-common.html

Getachew, A. (2008). Epidemiology of gallstone disease in Gondar university hospital, as seen in the department of radiology. *Ethiopian Journal of Health Development*, 22(2). Retrieved from http://ejhd.uib.no/ejhd-v22-n2/206%20Epidemiology%20of%20gallstone%20disease%20in%20Gondar%20University%20H.pdf

# REFERENCES

Howenstein, J. (2007 Dec.3). Bile salts can heal psoriasis, septicemia, viral infections, and excess estrogen. *NewsWithViews.com*. Retrieved from http://www.newswithviews.com/Howenstine/james63.htm

Johns Hopkins Medicine (2001). Gallstone disease: introduction. Retrieved from http://www.hopkinsmedicine.org/gastroenterology_hepatology/_pdfs/pancreas_biliary_tract/gallstone_disease.pdf

Méndez-Sánchez, N., Chavez-Tapia, N., Motola-Kuba, D. & Sanchez-Lara, K. (2005).

Metabolic syndrome as a risk factor for gallstone disease. *World Journal of Gastroenterology* 11, 1653–1657.

## Chapter 23: One Very Interesting Year

Moritz, A. (2007). *The Liver and Gallbladder Miracle Cleanse: An All-Natural, At-Home Flush to Purify and Rejuvenate Your Body.* Ener-chi.com: North Carolina.

## Chapter 24: The Undiplomatic Breakthrough

Shukla, V. & Prakash, A. (1998). Biliary heavy metal concentrations in carcinoma of the gallbladder: case-control study. *British Medical Journal*, 317:1288. doi: 1998;317:1288

Sipos, P., et al. (2003). Some effects of lead contamination on liver and gallbladder bile. *Chemical Research Center, Hungarian Academy of Science, Semmelweis University, Budapest*, 47(1–4):139–142.

Retrieved from
http://www2.sci.u-szeged.hu/ABS/2003/ActaHP/47139.pdf

Srisukho, S., et al. (1996). Mercury content in the gallstones and bile of Thai people (Chiang Mai and Bangkok) and Japanese. *Journal of the Medical Association of Thailand,* 79(5), 299-308. Retrieved from http://www.ncbi.nlm.nih.gov/pubmed/8708522

## Chapter 26: What Comes Out Goes Around

Patrick, L. (2002). Mercury toxicity and antioxidants: Part I: Role of glutathione and alpha-lipoic acid in the treatment of mercury toxicity. *Alternative Medicine Review,* 7(6): 456–471. Retrieved from http://www.altmedrev.com/publications/7/6/456.pdf

## Chapter 27: Crisis of Healing

Mercola, J. & Klinghardt, D. (2001). Mercury toxicity and systemic elimination agents. *Journal of Nutritional & Environmental Medicine.* (11):53–62. Retrieved from http://www.biblelife.org/Mercury-toxicity-Dr-Klinghardt.pdf

Murray, A. & Kidby, D. (1975). Subcellular location of mercury in yeast grown in the presence of mercuric chloride. *Journal of General Microbiology.* (86):66–74. Retrieved from http://mic.sgmjournals.org/content/86/1/66.full.pdf+html

## Chapter 29: Human Canary

Institute for Agriculture and Trade Policy. (2009, Jan. 28). Study finds high-fructose corn syrup contains mercury. *The Washington Post.*

Retrieved from http://www.washingtonpost.com/wp-dyn/content/article/2009/01/26/AR2009012601831.html

## Chapter 30: The Ancient Remedy

Dinsley, J. (2006). *Charcoal Remedies.Com. The Complete Handbook of Medicinal Charcoal and Its Applications.* GateKeepers Book.

## Chapter 31: The Unexpected Hormonal Connection

Brownlee, K., Moore, A., & Hackney, A. (2005). Relationship between circulating cortisol and testosterone: influence of physical exercise. *Journal of Sports Science & Medicine* 4(1):76–83. Retrieved from http://www.ncbi.nlm.nih.gov/pubmed/24431964

Haley, B. (2005). Mercury toxicity: genetic susceptibility, and synergistic effects. *Medical Veritas,* 2:535–542. Retrieved from http://homeoint.ru/pdfs/haley.pdf

## Chapter 32: Convergence

Barbagallo, M., et al. (1999). Effects of glutathione on red blood cell intracellular magnesium: relation to glucose metabolism. *Hypertension,* 34:76–82. Retrieved from http://hyper.ahajournals.org/content/34/1/76.full.pdf+html

Goldman, M. & Blackburn, P. (1979). The effect of mercuric chloride on thyroid function in the rat. *Toxicology and Applied Pharmacology* 48(1):49–55. Retrieved from http://www.sciencedirect.com/science/article/pii/S0041008X79800071

Inkinen, J., et al. (2001). Direct effect of thyroxine on pig sphincter of Oddi contractility. *Digestive Diseases and Sciences,* 46(1), 182–186. Retrieved from http://link.springer.com/article/10.1023/A:1005674211976#page-1

Sugiura, Y., Tamai, Y., & Tanaka, H. (1978). Selenium protection against mercury toxicity: high binding affinity of methylmercury by selenium-containing ligands in comparison with sulfur-containing ligands. *Bioinorganic Chemistry* 9(2): 167–180. Retrieved from http://www.sciencedirect.com/science/article/pii/S0006306100802884

Trautwein, E. & Hayes, K. (1994). Thyroxine and propylthiouracil supplements reduce lithogenic index and cholesterol gallstones in hamsters. *The Journal of Nutritional Biochemistry,* 5(8):397–405. Retrieved from http://www.sciencedirect.com/science/article/pii/0955286394900582

Vassilakis, J. & Nicolopoulos, N. (1981). Dissolution of gallstones following thyroxine administration. A case report. *Hepato-gastroenterology,* 28(1):60–61. Retrieved from http://europepmc.org/abstract/MED/6894289/reload=0;jsessionid=dmGG5UKUxWDyUrOezjIk.12

Völzke, H., Robinson, D., & Ulrich, J. (2005). Association between thyroid function and gallstone disease. *World Journal of Gastroenterology* 11(35):5530–5534. Retrieved from http://www.wjgnet.com/1007-9327/11/5530.pdf?origin=publication_detail

Wu, P. (2000). Thyroid disease and diabetes. *Clinical Diabetes* 18(1). Retrieved from http://journal.diabetes.org/clinicaldiabetes/v18n12000/pg38.htm

**Chapter 33: Thyroid Reboot**

Brownstein, D. (2009). *Iodine: Why You Need It, Why You Can't Live without It.* (4th ed.). West Bloomfield, MI: Medical Alternative Press.

Ertek, S., Cicero, A., Caglar, O., & Erdogan, G. (2010). Relationship between serum zinc levels, thyroid hormones and thyroid volume following successful iodine supplementation. *Hormones* 9(3):263–268. Retrieved from http://www.hormones.gr/pdf/HORMONES%202010%20263-268.pdf

Köhrle, J. (2000). The deiodinase family: selenoenzymes regulating thyroid hormone availability and action. *Cellular and Molecular Life Sciences* 57(13–14): 1853–1863. Retrieved from http://www.ncbi.nlm.nih.gov/pubmed/11215512

Köhrle, J., Oertel, M. & Gross, M. (1992). Selenium supply regulates thyroid function, thyroid hormone synthesis and metabolism by altering the expression of selenoenzymes Type I 5'-deiodinase and glutathione peroxidase. *Thyridology* 4(1):17–21. Retrieved from http://www.ncbi.nlm.nih.gov/pubmed/1284327

Morell, S. (2009). The great iodine debate. The Weston A. Price
    Foundation. Retrieved from
    http://www.westonaprice.org/metabolic-disorders/the-great-
    iodine-debate

Ruz, E., et al. (1999). Single and multiple selenium-zinc-iodine
    deficiencies affect rat thyroid metabolism and ultrastructure. *The
    Journal of Nutrition,* 129(1):174–180. Retrieved from
    http://jn.nutrition.org/content/129/1/174.short

Sircus, M. (2007). Iodine and chelation. *International Veritas Medical
    Association.* Retrieved from
    http://www.alkalizeforhealth.net/Liodine2.htm

Zimmermann, M., & Kohrle, J. (2002). The impact of iron and selenium
    deficiencies on iodine and thyroid metabolism: biochemistry and
    relevance to public health. *Thyroid: Official Journal of the American
    Thyroid Association.* 12(10):867–878. Retrieved from
    http://www.ncbi.nlm.nih.gov/pubmed/12487769

## Chapter 34: The Supplanting Agents

Abraham, G. (2005). The historical background of the iodine project. *The
    Original Internist.* Summer: 57–66. Retrieved from
    http://www.optimox.com/pics/Iodine/pdfs/IOD08.pdf

Cann, S., van Netten, J., & van Netten, C. (2000). Hypothesis: iodine,
    selenium, and the development of breast cancer. *Cancer Causes and
    Control,* 11:121–127. Retrieved from
    http://link.springer.com/article/10.1023/
    A:1008925301459#page-1

# REFERENCES

Brownstein, D. (2005). Orthosupplementation. *The Original Internist.* 12(3):105–108. Retrieved from http://iodineresearch.com/orthobrownstien.html

Feldkamp, J., et al. (1999). Fas-mediated apoptosis is inhibited by TSH and iodine in moderate concentrations in primary human thyrocytes in vitro. *Hormone and Metabolic Research,* 31(6):355–358. Retrieved from https://www.thieme-connect.com/products/ejournals/abstract/10.1055/s-2007-978753

Jensen, B. & Anderson, M. (1973). *Empty Harvest.* New York, NY: Penguin Putnam.

Mercola, J. (2009). Avoid this if you want to keep your thyroid healthy. Retrieved from http://articles.mercola.com/sites/articles/archive/2009/09/05/Another-Poison-Hiding-in-Your-Environment.aspx

Patrick, L. (2008). Iodine: deficiency and therapeutic considerations. *Alternative Medicine Review*, 13(2):116–127. Retrieved from http://web.a.ebscohost.com/abstract?direct=true&profile=ehost&scope=site&authtype=crawler&jrnl=10895159&AN=33337826&h=6PjaZtsF04kxnLvXiKMOIvA2JdbPL3998uLm2t8%2fJQinGknfiOTXjtsMjKptuMKPICMUhBDsSBov7MKFKni2zA%3d%3d&crl=c

Piccone, N. (2011). The silent epidemic of iodine deficiency. *Life Extension Magazine*, October. Retrieved from http://www.lef.org/magazine/mag2011/oct2011_The-Silent-Epidemic-of-Iodine-Deficiency_01.htm

Power, L. (2006). Iodine & thyroid deficiencies: linked to thyroid and breast cancer, fibrocystic breast disease, infertility, obesity, mental retardation & halide toxemia. Retrieved from http://www.laurapower.com/page26.html

Showler, L. Iodine deficiency and the endocrine system. Retrieved from http://www.livingnaturally.com/PDFDocs/e/E0KE5CTEDA6D8JML5SXJNNL1LMVJ9C42.PDF

Vitti, P., et al. (2003). Europe is iodine deficient. *The Lancelot.* (361):1226. Retrieved from http://download.thelancet.com/pdfs/journals/lancet/PIIS0140673603129352.pdf

Kurokawa, Y., et al. (1990). Toxicity and carcinogenicity of potassium bromate—a new renal carcinogen. *Environmental Health Perspectives.* July (87):309–335. Retrieved from http://www.ncbi.nlm.nih.gov/pmc/articles/PMC1567851/

World Health Organization (2007). Iodine deficiency in Europe: A continuing public health problem. *WHO.* Retrieved from http://www.who.int/nutrition/publications/VMNIS_Iodine_deficiency_in_Europe.pdf

## Chapter 36: Not a Chance

Camargo, R., et al. (2008). Thyroid and the environment: exposure to excessive nutritional iodine increases the prevalence of thyroid disorders in São Paulo, Brazil. *European Journal of Endocrinology.* 159:293–299. Retrieved from http://www.eje.org/content/159/3/293.full.pdf+html

# REFERENCES

Fisk, M., et al. (2010). Asthma in swimmers: a review of the current literature. *The Physician and Sports Medicine.* 38(4):28–34. Retrieved from http://www.ncbi.nlm.nih.gov/pubmed/21150139

Sircus, M. (2011). Iodine phobia & salt truth. *International Veritas Medical Association.* Retrieved from http://drsircus.com/medicine/iodine/iodine-phobia-salt-truth#_ednref2

United States Environmental Protection Agency (1997). Research plan for microbial pathogens and disinfection byproducts in drinking water. Washington D.C. Government Printing Office. Retrieved from http://nepis.epa.gov/Exe/ZyPDF.cgi/30003KZW.PDF?Dockey=30003KZW.PDF

Zimmermann, M., et al. (2003). Thyroid size and goiter prevalence after introduction of iodized salt: a 5-year prospective study in schoolchildren in Côte d'Ivoire. *The American Journal of Clinical Nutrition.* 77:663–7. Retrieved from http://ajcn.nutrition.org/content/77/3/663.full.pdf+html

## Chapter 37: Different Problem, Same Solution

American Environmental Health Studies Project (2004). *The Fluoride Deception.* Retrieved from https://www.youtube.com/watch?v=eBZRb-73tLc

Bryson, C. (2004). *The Fluoride Deception.* New York, NY: Seven Stories Press.

## Chapter 38: Dipping Seven Times in the Jordan

Berger, J., Redinger, R., & Small, D. (1970). Instrument for sampling and measuring bile flow. *Medical & Biological Engineering & Computing.* 8(1):19–24. Retrieved from http://link.springer.com/article/10.1007%2FBF02551745

Howenstein, J. (2007 Dec.3). Bile salts can heal psoriasis, septicemia, viral infections, and excess estrogen. *NewsWithViews.com.* Retrieved from http://www.newswithviews.com/Howenstine/james63.htm

## Chapter 39: From Parasitic to Symbiotic

Absar, A., et al. (2010). The global war against intestinal parasites—should we use a holistic approach? *International Journal of Infectious Diseases.* 14:732–738. doi:10.1016/j.ijid.2009.11.036

Aldenborg, F., Fall, M, & Enerback, L. (1986). Proliferation and transepithelial migration of mucosal mast cells in interstitial cystitis. *Immunology.* 58:411–416. Retrieved from http://www.ncbi.nlm.nih.gov/pmc/articles/PMC1453481/

Bethony, J., et al. (2006). Soil-transmitted helminth infections: ascariasis, trichuriasis, and hookworm. *The Lance.com.* May 6. 367:1521–1532. Retrieved from http://140.226.65.22/Davis_lab/Parasit_links/Soil_Transmitted_%20Helminths_Lancet_%20'06.pdf

Cook, G. (1994). Enterobius vermicularis infection. *GUT.* 35(9):1159–1162. Retrieved from http://www.ncbi.nlm.nih.gov/pmc/articles/PMC1375686/

# REFERENCES

Boroch, A. (2008). *The Candida Cure. Yeast, Fungus, & Your Health*. Los Angeles, CA: Quintessential Healing Publishing, Inc.

Basuroy, S., et al. (2005). Acetaldehyde disrupts tight junctions and adherens junctions in human colonic mucosa: protection by EGF and L-glutamine. *American Journal of Physiology*. Aug; 289(2): G367-75. Retrieved from http://www.ncbi.nlm.nih.gov/pubmed/15718285

Liao, K., et al. (1992). Improved postfixation treatment of glutaraldehyde fixed porcine aortic valves by monosodium glutamate. *Artificial Organs*. 16(3):267–272. Retrieved from http://www.ncbi.nlm.nih.gov/pubmed/10078257

Clark, H. (1996). How parasites causes cancer and HIV. *The Light Party*. Retrieved from http://www.lightparty.com/Health/PARASITE.html

Crompton, D. (1984). *Parasites and people*. London, England. Macmillan Publishers, Ltd.

Crompton, D. & Savioli, L. (1993). Intestinal parasitic infections and urbanization. *Bulletin of the World Health Organization*. 71(1):1–7. Retrieved from http://apps.who.int/iris/handle/10665/49956

Duval-Araujo, I., et al. (2007). Bacterial colonization of the ileum in rats with obstructive jaundice. *Brazilian Journal of Microbiology*. 38:406–408. Retrieved from http://www.scielo.br/scielo.php?pid=S1517-83822007000300003&script=sci_arttext

Eamonn, M., et al. (2006). Small intestinal bacterial overgrowth: roles of antibiotics, prebiotics, and probiotics. *Gastroenterology.* 130:578–590. Retrieved from http://www.med.upenn.edu/gastro/documents/Gastroenterologybacterialovergrowth.pdf

Ehrlich, S. (2012). Internal parasites. *Complementary and Alternative Medicine Guide, University of Maryland Medical Center.* Retrieved from http://umm.edu/health/medical/altmed/condition/intestinal-parasites

Geier, D., et al. (2009). A prospective study of prenatal mercury exposure from maternal dental amalgams and autism severity. *Acta Neurobiologiae Experimentalis.* 69(2):189–197. Retrieved from http://www.ncbi.nlm.nih.gov/pubmed/19593333

Ingram, C. (2008). *The Cure Is in the Cupboard: How to Use Oregano for Better Health*. Vernon Hills, IL: Knowledge House Products.

Miroff, G., et al. (1991). Molybdenum for Candida albicans patients and other problems. *The Digest of Chiropractic Economics.* 31(4):56–63. Retrieved from http://www.arthritistrust.org/wp-content/uploads/2013/03/Molybdenum-for-Candida-albicans-Patients.pdf

Nieminen, M., et al. (2009). Acetaldehyde production from ethanol and glucose by non-Candida albicans yeasts in vitro. *Oral Oncology.* 45(12):245–248. Retrieved from http://www.oraloncology.com/article/S1368-8375(09)00879-3/fulltext

# REFERENCES

Price, W. (2003). *Nutrition and Physical Degeneration* (6th ed.). New Canaan, CT: Keats Publishing.

Quihui-Cota, L. & Morales-Figueroa, G. (2012). Persistence of intestinal parasitic infections during the national de-worming campaign in schoolchildren of northwestern Mexico: a cross-sectional study. *Annals of Gastroenterology.* 25:57–60. Retrieved from http://www.scirp.org/journal/PaperInformation.aspx?PaperID=30609#.U1alwvldWSo

Schmidt, G. & Roberts, L. (2000). *Foundations of Parasitology* (6th ed.). New York, NY: McGraw- Hill Publishing. Retrieved from http://www.uni-bielefeld.de/biologie/Didaktik/Zoologie/html_deutsch/pics/Trematoda.pdf

Stepek, G., et al. (2006). Human gastrointestinal nematode infections: Are new control methods required? *International Journal of Experimental Pathology.* 87(5):325–341. Retrieved from http://www.ncbi.nlm.nih.gov/pmc/articles/PMC2517378/

Truss, C., et al. (1984). Metabolic abnormalities in patients with chronic candidiasis. The acetaldehyde hypothesis. *Journal of Orthomolecular Psychiatry.* 13(2):66–93. Retrieved from http://www.orthomolecular.org/library/jom/1984/pdf/1984-v13n02-p066.pdf

Uittamo, J., et al. (2009). Chronic candidosis and oral cancer in APECED-patients: Production of carcinogenic acetaldehyde from glucose and ethanol by Candida albicans. *International Journal of Cancer.* 124:754–756. Retrieved from http://onlinelibrary.wiley.com/doi/10.1002/ijc.23976/pdf

United States Department of Health and Human Services (2012). Giardiasis surveillance United States, 2009–2010. Retrieved from http://www.cdc.gov/mmwr/preview/mmwrhtml/ss6105a2.htm

United States Department of Health and Human Services (2013). DPDx-laboratory identification of parasitic diseases of public health concern. Retrieved from http://www.cdc.gov/dpdx/diagnosticProcedures/index.html

United States Environmental Protection Agency (2000). Acetaldehyde 75-07-0 hazard summary. Retrieved from http://www.epa.gov/ttn/atw/hlthef/acetalde.html

United States Environmental Protection Agency (1999). Giardia: drinking water health advisory. Retrieved from http://water.epa.gov/action/advisories/drinking/upload/2009_02_03_criteria_humanhealth_microbial_giardiaha.pdf

Walker, M. (1997). *Olive Leaf Extract*. New York, NY: Kensington Publications.

Weintraub, S. (1998). *The Parasite Menace*. Pleasant Grove, UT: Woodland Publishing.

Wondro: The famous herbal remedy inside out. Retrieved from http://www.scribd.com/doc/101099776/Wondro-Inside-Out

World Health Organization (2012). Research priorities for Helminth infections. Retrieved from http://apps.who.int/iris/bitstream/10665/75922/1/WHO_TRS_972_eng.pdf

Zaidel, O., & Lin, H. (2003). Uninvited guests: the impact of small intestinal bacterial overgrowth on nutritional status. *Nutritional Issues in Gastroenterology.* July:27–34. Retrieved from http://www.medicine.virginia.edu/clinical/departments/medicine/divisions/digestive-health/nutrition-support-team/nutrition-articles/zaidelarticle.pdf

## Chapter 40: Welcome To Your Life

Davis, W. (2007). Is your bottled water killing you? Health benefits of magnesium replacement. *Life Extension Magazine.* February. Retrieved from http://www.lef.org/magazine/mag2007/feb2007_report_water_02.htm

Hyman, M. (2012). Magnesium: meet the most powerful relaxation mineral available. *Drhyman.com.* March, 19. Retrieved from http://drhyman.com/blog/2010/05/20/magnesium-the-most-powerful-relaxation-mineral-available/

Johnson, S. (2001). The multifaceted and widespread pathology of magnesium deficiency. *Medical Hypotheses.* 56(2):163–170. Retrieved from http://www.naturaleater.com/science-articles/The-multifaceted-and-widespread-pathology-of-magnesium-deficiency.pdf

Sircus, M. (2009). Magnesium and cell survival (Glutathione). *International Medical Veritas Association.* December. Retrieved from http://drsircus.com/medicine/magnesium/magnesium-and-cell-survival-glutathione

Tong, G., & Rude, K. (2005). Magnesium deficiency in critical illness. *Journal of Intensive Care Medicine.* Jan-Feb: 20(1):3–17. Retrieved from http://www.ncbi.nlm.nih.gov/pubmed/15665255

Printed in Great Britain
by Amazon.co.uk, Ltd.,
Marston Gate.